Government Size and Implications for Economic Growth

Government Size and Implications for Economic Growth

Andreas Bergh and Magnus Henrekson

The AEI Press

Publisher for the American Enterprise Institute

WASHINGTON, D.C.

Distributed by arrangement with the Rowman & Littlefield Publishing Group, 4501 Forbes Boulevard, Suite 200, Lanham, Maryland 20706. To order call toll free 1-800-462-6420 or 1-717-794-3800. For all other inquiries please contact AEI Press, 1150 Seventeenth Street, N.W. Washington, D.C. 20036 or call 1-800-862-5801.

NRI NATIONAL RESEARCH INITIATIVE

This publication is a project of the National Research Initiative, a program of the American Enterprise Institute that is designed to support, publish, and disseminate research by university-based scholars and other independent researchers who are engaged in the exploration of important public policy issues.

Library of Congress Cataloging-in-Publication Data

Bergh, Andreas.
   Government size and implications for economic growth / Andreas Bergh and Magnus Henrekson.
      p. cm.
   Includes bibliographical references.
   ISBN-13: 978-0-8447-4327-1 (cloth)
   ISBN-10: 0-8447-4327-5 (cloth)
   ISBN-13: 978-0-8447-4353-0 (pbk.)
   ISBN-10: 0-8447-4353-4 (pbk.)
   [etc.]
   1. Expenditures, Public. 2. Economic development. 3. Taxation. I. Henrekson, Magnus. II. Title.

HJ7461.B47 2010
338.9—dc22

                                                          2010009573

14 13 12 11 10   1 2 3 4 5 6 7

Printed in the United States of America

Contents

List of Illustrations

Acknowledgment

The authors thank Daniel Hedblom for excellent research assistance.

Introduction:
Why Growth Is Important, and
Why Government Size May Matter

The debate regarding the relationship between government size and economic development has been intense for decades. The state of research is seemingly contradictory, with some scholars arguing that big government decreases growth, and some declaring this not to be the case.

A close look at the literature reveals that results are not as conflicting as they may at first appear. Different researchers have used different measures of growth and of government size, and they have studied different types of countries. When we focus on studies that examine growth of real gross domestic product (GDP) per capita over longer time periods, the research is actually close to a consensus: In rich countries, there is a negative correlation between total size of government and growth.

To arrive at this conclusion, we have reviewed a wide body of literature on the subject. Here we describe the state of research and discuss what findings can be trusted, as well as the most important policy implications of those findings. But first, some words on why the issue itself is important.

The growth effects of government size are crucial, both in countries with relatively small governments, such as the United States, and in countries like Sweden, where government spending exceeds 50 percent of GDP. From one year to the next, the difference between annual economic growth at 2 percent or 2.5 percent is important enough, since it means several billions of dollars, more or less, in the hands of both households and politicians. From a longer perspective, the level of annual growth of GDP per capita is even more important: It ultimately determines which countries will grow rich and which will become or remain relatively poor.

As shown in figure I-1, an annual growth rate of 2 percent means that the economic standard of living doubles in thirty-six years. But if the annual

1

FIGURE I-1

THE VALUE OF AN INITIAL INVESTMENT OF $1,000 WITH ANNUAL
GROWTH AT 2 OR 3 PERCENT

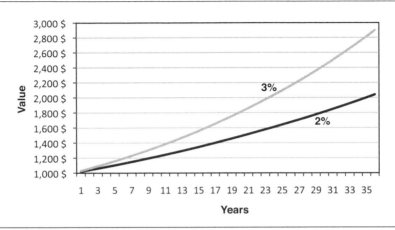

SOURCE: Authors' illustration.

growth is instead 3 percent, a doubling of the standard of living takes a mere twenty-four years.

Focusing policy on economic growth and standard of living may seem narrow-mindedly materialistic to some. But growth is ultimately about becoming more efficient in getting what we want—including food, housing, and health care, as well as literature, arts, and leisure. It is hardly surprising, therefore, to find a strong positive correlation between GDP per capita and other measures of well-being, such as longevity and infant mortality, as demonstrated by Lant Pritchett and Lawrence Summers (1996) and visualized by Hans Rosling (2010) using statistics from the United Nations. Despite some claims to the contrary, a clear link also exists between income and happiness, as recently shown by Betsey Stevenson and Justin Wolfers (2008).

The misconception that growth is a materialistic concept probably comes from its typically being measured by looking only at GDP per capita. This measures economic activity in the formal sector of the economy without taking into account how many hours are actually worked. For example, Schmid (2008) shows that the United States is about 30 percent richer than

Sweden—but that approximately half of the difference can be explained by the fact that Swedes work fewer hours with respect to market work.

The question is, how do we know if Swedes work fewer hours because they simply prefer leisure more than Americans do, or because they must pay much higher taxes when they work? The answer is suggested by the greater number of hours Swedes spend on unpaid household work as compared to Americans. If Swedes simply liked leisure more than Americans do, they would, presumably, work less than Americans both on the market and in the household. The greater amount of time they spend on unpaid household work strongly implies that taxes are part of the explanation. Taxes affect the choice between taxed market work and untaxed household work or leisure. When taxes are high, market work pays less, and leisure and household work become more attractive.[1] In the standard neoclassical growth model, this affects only the level of income and not its growth rate. But when services are provided by professionals, incentives emerge to invest in new knowledge, to develop more effective tools and superior contractual arrangements, and to create more flexible organizational structures. Thus, higher rates of personal taxation reduce the scope for entrepreneurial expansion into new market activities that economize on time use or supply close substitutes for home-produced services. And without the emergence of new service jobs replacing traditional manufacturing jobs, the demand for tax-financed transfers increases. This puts an upward pressure on the tax and expenditure ratios, which provides an additional channel resulting in slower economic growth.

When discussing taxes, it is important not to confuse marginal tax rates with average taxes. The marginal tax (for income) is the tax rate applied to an additional dollar earned. In progressive tax systems, the marginal tax rate may well be much higher than the average tax. For a single person deciding whether to work or not, the marginal tax rate is the important factor—it determines how much income he or she will earn from working an extra hour. But when describing the total size of the public sector, a better measure is the tax ratio: the sum of all public tax revenue divided by GDP.

To illustrate, figure I-2 shows top marginal income tax rates in Sweden and the United States, and figure I-3 shows total taxes as a share of GDP.

In the 1970s, marginal taxes were higher than they are today in most industrialized countries. In fact, as shown in figure I-2, the top marginal tax rate was actually higher for some U.S. household types in the early 1970s

FIGURE I-2

TOP MARGINAL INCOME TAX RATE IN SWEDEN AND THE UNITED STATES, 1970–2003

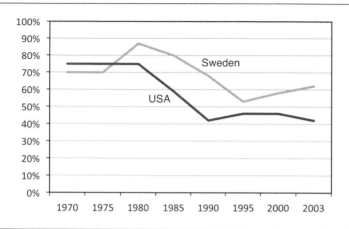

SOURCE: Economic Freedom Index (Gwartney et al. [2008]).
NOTE: The difference in actual taxation is underestimated for three reasons: 1) In the United States, the highest rate kicks in at a higher income; 2) in the United States, lower marginal tax rates apply for several household types; 3) in Sweden, mandatory employer fees add substantially to the total tax wedge.

than it was in Sweden. Around 1980, the marginal tax rate for a well-paid Swedish white-collar worker peaked at 87 percent. Since then, however, marginal tax rates have fallen in both Sweden and the United States, as well as in most other Western countries. The decrease has been sharper in the United States than in Sweden, and, as a matter of fact, figure I-2 underestimates the difference for several reasons. In Sweden, payroll taxes are substantial, and many middle-income earners face high marginal taxes, and in the United States, many household types face a lower marginal tax than the highest one shown in figure I-2. Finally, it is important to remember that the level of total taxation has been much lower in the United States than in Sweden since 1960, as shown in figure I-3.

Simple comparisons of Sweden and the United States are useful illustrations of different types of tax policy, but they do not prove anything regarding the relationship between economic growth and (the level and structure of) taxes. To know more, we need to consider more countries and other factors systematically. The good news is that this is exactly what modern

FIGURE I-3

TAXES AS A SHARE OF GDP IN SWEDEN AND THE UNITED STATES,
1925–2007

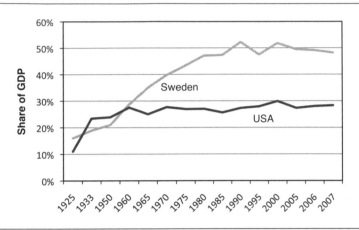

SOURCE: Rodriguez (1981) and new data from SourceOECD.

empirical research in economics is about, and for a long time a great deal of effort has been devoted to examining the link between government size and economic growth.

In the analysis presented here, we probe deeper into the debate by reviewing the most recent economic research on growth and government size. Our conclusions can be summarized as follows:

- While results vary, depending on scientific method and the countries studied, the most recent studies of high scientific quality typically find a negative correlation between government size and economic growth in rich countries.

- Looking closely at what governments actually do and how they finance their activities reveals that different activities have different effects on growth. Thus, in addition to government size, what governments do and how this is financed matter.

- Research has recently identified institutions as a crucial determinant of economic growth. Property rights, a noncorrupt legal system, and economic openness seem particularly important for growth.

- The Scandinavian welfare states have done reasonably well in terms of growth during the last ten to twelve years, not because of, but rather despite, having big government sectors. In many areas, these countries offset the negative effect of large governments by applying market-friendly policies in other areas, such as trade openness and inflation control.

Currently, research is still struggling with some important questions: How have the Scandinavian welfare states managed to combine market-friendly policies with big governments? Can the direction of causality between government size and growth be established? We do not claim to have the definitive answers to these questions, but we will introduce the reader to our interpretations of the most recent research.

The remainder of this essay is organized as follows. In chapter 1 we briefly survey the literature regarding theoretical reasons for expecting government size to affect growth. In chapter 2, we take a closer look at the empirical evidence by describing different types of studies that have examined the relationship between government size and economic growth. We also survey some of the recent research on the growth effects of institutional quality in general and economic freedom in particular. This leads directly to chapter 3, which explores the interesting fact that several of the countries that have increased their degree of economic freedom substantially are ones with large public sectors. In chapter 4 we discuss why high rates of personal taxation induce consumers to produce personal services themselves. As a consequence, higher rates of personal taxation reduce the scope for entrepreneurial expansion into new market activities that economize on time use or supply close substitutes for home-produced services. With less scope for division of labor, economic growth is likely to be impaired. Finally, we summarize our main conclusions and discuss their policy implications.

1

How Do We Know If Big Government Is Good or Bad for Growth?

The question we tackle here is a controversial one. It is easy for anyone to produce seemingly clear evidence that big government decreases growth, and it is equally easy for those holding the opposite view to produce graphs that point in the opposite direction. In this chapter we illustrate this by showing that seemingly clear evidence is often insufficient to settle the issue. We also show that there are theoretical mechanisms working in both directions, i.e., there are some reasons why government may be bad for growth but there are also reasons why the effect might be positive.[1] Thus, sophisticated empirical methods are needed to settle the question.

Why Seemingly Clear Evidence May Be Insufficient

The scatter plot in figure 1-1 shows annual pairs of growth in real GDP per capita and government size (measured as taxes as a share of GDP) for countries in the Organisation for Economic Co-operation and Development (OECD) during the period 1970–2005. A weak negative correlation suggests that countries with larger governments on average experience slower growth.

On the other hand, the picture is far from unequivocal. A number of countries with a disastrous growth record have had very low taxes (such as Portugal and Greece in the mid-1970s), and several with very high taxes have experienced years with very high growth. If, for some reason, you believed that big government impedes growth only if you want to achieve very high rates of growth, you could back this assertion simply by excluding observations of annual growth rates exceeding 6 percent; this is shown in figure 1-2.

FIGURE 1-1

CROSS-COUNTRY CORRELATION BETWEEN GROWTH AND GOVERNMENT SIZE MEASURED AS TAX REVENUE OVER GDP, ANNUAL PAIRS, OECD 1970–2005

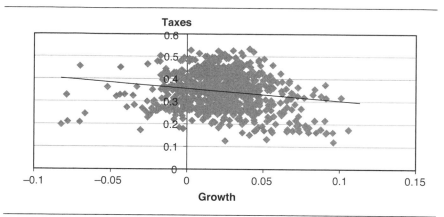

SOURCE: Authors' calculations based on data in Bergh and Karlsson (2010).

FIGURE 1-2

CROSS-COUNTRY CORRELATION BETWEEN GROWTH AND GOVERNMENT SIZE, EXCLUDING COUNTRIES WITH ANNUAL GROWTH EXCEEDING 6 PERCENT, OECD 1970–2005

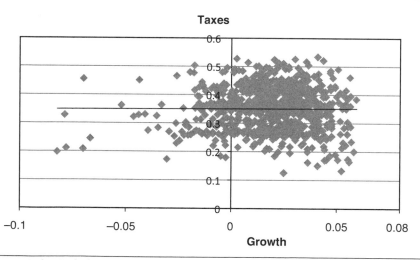

SOURCE: Authors' calculations based on data in Bergh and Karlsson (2010).

FIGURE 1-3

CROSS-COUNTRY CORRELATION BETWEEN GROWTH AND GOVERNMENT
SIZE USING AVERAGES OVER DECADES RATHER THAN ANNUAL VALUES
OF GROWTH AND GOVERNMENT SIZE, OECD, 1970–2005

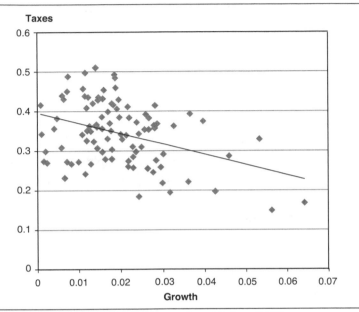

SOURCE: Authors' calculations based on data in Bergh and Karlsson (2010).

If, on the other hand, you believed that government size affects growth through mechanisms that take more than a year to materialize, you might instead want to plot growth and government size averaged over longer time periods—decades, for example. In figure 1-3, we plot average growth for the 1970s, 1980s, 1990s, and 2000–2005 against average government size in the respective periods. This change actually strengthens the negative correlation: No OECD country has collected taxes of more than 40 percent of GDP *and* during the same decade achieved an average annual growth rate exceeding 3 percent. There is a great deal of variation in both tax ratios and growth rates, but the negative correlation between the two is obvious (and statistically significant).

For several reasons, however, the seemingly unambiguous relationship in figure 1-3 is not evidence of a negative effect of government size on economic growth. We have already seen that annual data can give a different picture than averages of longer time periods, and we have seen that a correlation may be sensitive to the exclusion of some observations. Several additional aspects require attention in our case.

First of all, the pattern may change if we measure government size differently. Should we use taxes, expenditure, the share of government employees relative to total employment, or some other measure of government size?

Second, the result may depend on the selection of countries examined. In fact, the negative relationship in figure 1-3 is largely driven by a small number of countries with small government sectors and rapid growth, such as South Korea and Ireland. If these countries were excluded from the sample, the pattern, while still visible, would be less clear cut. On the other hand, the OECD countries are not a random sample of rich countries; to the contrary, they are united by their commitment to democracy and to a liberal market economic system, working explicitly to boost growth and living standards. Adding a number of rich, non-OECD countries to the sample again might change the picture.

Third, the observed relationship may be played out through several omitted variables. Notably, a large proportion of elderly people in the population will lower the rate of growth and increase the relative size of government through the financing of health care and pensions. As a result, high taxes and slow growth will go together (exhibiting a positive correlation) not because one causes the other, but because demography causes both!

Another important factor that needs to be taken into account is the so-called catching-up effect: Poor countries can more easily increase their rate of growth than rich ones by learning from the rich countries' mistakes and adopting technologies already developed and used there.[2]

A fourth problem is that, even when other explanatory factors (such as demography and initial GDP) are taken into account, it is far from clear that the relationship between government size and growth can be given a *causal* interpretation. As we will see, there are some reasons to believe that countries grow more slowly on average because they have larger governments. But, in a strict statistical sense, it is equally possible that those that grow more slowly tend to let their governments grow relatively larger.

Yet another difficulty in establishing causality is that when a country increases taxes and experiences problems as a result, it is likely to lower the taxes again. On the other hand, countries that do not experience problems are more likely to retain high taxes. If this is the case, statistical analyses are likely to suggest no relationship between taxes and economic growth. But if countries with low levels of taxation decide to raise taxes, they will still run into trouble!

In short, four fundamental problems must be confronted in studies like these:

- The measurement problem: How do we properly measure government size?

- The sample selection problem: What countries should we study, and during what period of time?

- The model selection problem: What other variables should we include in the analysis?

- The causality problem: How do we know if government size causes economic outcomes, and not the other way around?

Accounting for these problems is a difficult task, but not an entirely intractable one. By gathering and comparing results from several studies that look at different groups of countries across different time periods using a variety of statistical techniques, we obtain a clearer picture. Importantly, empirical studies must be complemented with careful theoretical reasoning to interpret the results.

The first three problems are easier to handle than the fourth. By examining research that has tested the relationship between government size and growth using different measures of government size, different time periods, and different countries in their samples, we know quite a bit about how these choices affect the results. A large literature also identifies the factors significantly related to growth and examines their relative importance.

A particularly important advance in social science research technology is the increased use of so-called panel data. This means that results do not rely only on comparisons among different countries at a certain point in time. Rather, panel data allow us to draw conclusions based on changes within countries over time, in addition to what can be inferred from differences across countries.

Why are panel data often preferable? Well, the number of factors that differ among countries is, of course, infinite. For example, Sweden is different from the United States not only in its having higher taxes, but in thousands of other dimensions as well. Even with the inclusion of factors such as the dependency ratio and initial GDP in the analysis, thousands of other omitted factors might still explain any growth difference in the data. Using panel data makes possible the assumption that these other factors that differentiate Sweden from the United States are constant over time. If this is at least approximately true, one can isolate the effect of the variables of interest, relying on variations within countries over time.

Having seen that the empirical evidence often turns out to be less clear-cut than it initially appears, we will now deal with our key question from a different angle: the theoretical one. Why would we expect any growth differences between countries with big and small governments?

Theoretical Expectations: Should We Expect Big Government To Be Good or Bad for Growth?

Do we expect countries with larger government sectors to grow faster or more slowly than those with small government sectors? What makes us think that government size should have any effect on economic growth at all?

The answer depends on how we look upon economic growth, and also on exactly how growth is defined. Over time, economists have accumulated knowledge regarding what explains growth, and three main perspectives can be identified:

- Neoclassical growth models

- Endogenous growth theory

- Focus on institutions as fundamental determinants of growth

In early so-called neoclassical growth models, the equilibrium growth rate of per-capita GDP is completely determined by the rate of technological progress in the economy.[3] Policy can still affect growth by affecting the level of savings or the level of employment, but the result will only be temporary, as the economy moves from one equilibrium to the next.[4] The productivity of labor and capital is determined by factors outside of these models.

In the more recent so-called endogenous growth theory policy, variables can have a permanent (long-run) effect on the equilibrium growth rate.[5] In these models, policy is important: Increased taxation may lead to permanently lower rates of growth, while a permanently higher level of productive government expenditure, such as on education or investment in infrastructure, may permanently increase the rate of economic growth. In other words, not only government size may matter for growth, but also how and on what tax revenue is being spent.

Currently, the buzzword of growth economics is "institutions" or "institutional quality." The idea is that certain types of economic arrangements, such as secure property rights and the rule of law, are particularly conducive to growth.[6] Clearly defined property rights and noncorrupt government are beneficial for more or less all types of economic activities, and the link between institutional quality and growth under these conditions is generally found to be very robust.

Importantly, these three different perspectives on growth do not contradict one another, but rather emphasize different aspects of the causes of growth. Furthermore, existing theories suggest several links between government size and growth, some negative and some positive. In the next section we list and describe these in more detail.

Arguments Pointing toward a Positive Link between Government Size and Growth

In this section we list four reasons why there may be a positive link between government size and growth. The idea is that there are things that governments do that are conducive to growth, and it is theoretically possible that these reasons are important also in rich countries.

Institutions. An important part of what government does is to uphold law and order. In particular, government can protect private property rights and punish those who violate contracts and agreements. Because well-protected property rights and the rule of law in general are essential for all sorts of investment, innovation, and trade, this aspect of government activity should be positively related to growth.

Market Failures. An extensive theoretical literature shows that, under some circumstances, free markets will fail to provide sufficient amounts of collective goods and goods with so-called positive externalities, and they may provide excessive amounts of goods with negative externalities. In both of these cases, government has an important role to play in filling societal needs. Furthermore, in the case of natural monopolies, public provision may be more efficient than private provision.

To get a flavor of these arguments, consider a good carrying a positive externality, such as education. On the market each person values education because of the private benefits it provides for him or her. But in addition to the private benefit, there may be a benefit for society as a whole in that, on average and with few exceptions, we become more productive when we deal with better-educated people—this is the positive externality. This argument might be true for research spending, as well as for basic education that increases literacy in society. Clearly, publicly supported education is important to the well-being of society.

On the other hand, some products have negative externalities, in that they harm people other than the consumer in a way that is not reflected in the market price. An example is cigarettes. The smoke imposes inconvenience and perhaps even inflicts harm on others besides the smoker him- or herself, who also does not bear fully the costs of the increased health expenditure and absenteeism incurred by the habit, especially not in redistributive welfare states. The theoretical implication is that taxation on cigarettes can be used to increase the market price so that it more accurately reflects the actual social cost of smoking.

In short, if substantial market failures make people less productive or generally unwilling to invest in some types of goods, larger government can, at least in theory, increase efficiency by correcting for such failure. Barr (1992) argues that substantial parts of the welfare state can, in fact, be motivated on efficiency grounds. Following Barro (1990), we can label public spending used to correct market failure "productive" government spending, possibly including spending on education, health care, and defense.

Social Inequality. Another important reason big government may be growth-promoting is that government spending and taxation can reduce the cost of social inequality. According to Myrdal (1960), social inequality impedes growth for at least two reasons: It leads to a waste of human capital as a consequence of poverty, and it restricts the opportunities for low-income individuals to exploit their talents. This idea has been further refined in "the social affinity theory" (Kristov et al. 1992), which predicts that government redistribution will be greater, the wider the pre-tax income gaps above median and the lower the gaps below median income. A greater government involvement in the economy can, in part, be aimed at reducing inequality.

Technical Arguments. In addition to the arguments based on institutions, market failure, and the costs of inequality, some statistical and technical factors might contribute to findings of a positive relationship between some measures of government size and economic growth. For example, in some studies, government goods and services are valued at their cost of production. This procedure gives rise to a number of difficulties that bias research results, due to the implicit assumptions that government output is produced with a constant-returns-to-scale technology, that all government production can be classified as final output rather than intermediate inputs lowering private sector production costs, and that the market value of government output is equal to the cost of production.[7]

Yet another factor to keep in mind is that both government consumption and investment are part of GDP when measured from the expenditure side. Thus, when these parts of government spending increase, GDP will increase by definition. In a way, explaining GDP growth by changes in government spending involves explaining something partly by itself. In particular, this problem lends an upward bias to the estimated effect during periods when the government spending share is increasing.

Finally, Kaldor (1966) claims that a high rate of utilization has a beneficial effect on long-run productivity growth. Insofar as an expansion of the public sector results in a higher utilization rate, there could be a positive effect on economic growth—a relationship known as Verdoorn's Law.

Arguments Pointing toward a Negative Effect

We now turn our attention to four reasons to expect a negative link between government size and growth. Importantly, even if government spending is conducive to growth, there are aspects of big government that unavoidably hamper economic activity and may thus lower growth.

Effect of Taxation. Taxation can affect growth in several ways. First of all, a tax may have a direct effect on GDP when it causes a distortion by introducing a wedge between supply and demand. In such a case, some transactions that would take place without the tax will not take place when the tax is levied. The result is the generation of neither tax revenue nor private surplus. This basic fact holds regardless of whether the buyer or the seller is the one legally required to pay the tax, and it holds regardless of whether the tax is introduced into a labor market, a capital market, or a market for consumption goods.

In models of endogenous growth, taxes may have a permanent effect on growth. For example, taxes that create a wedge between the gross and net returns on savings will lead to lower capital accumulation and, hence, a lower rate of economic growth.[8] Feldstein (2006) has pointed out that the (static) welfare costs of taxation are generated by the elasticity of taxable income with respect to tax rates, and that taxable income is probably more responsive than hours worked. In addition, dynamic efficiency losses are associated with occupational choice, schooling attainment, and other decisions that affect the accumulation of human capital.[9] For example, if the marginal tax rate is raised, a person might not only choose to work fewer hours, but might also turn down an offer for promotion, learn fewer new productive skills, take longer breaks, or work at a lower intensity. All these adjustments may be at least as important as working fewer hours in inducing a lowering of taxable income when the marginal tax rate is raised.

Crowding Out of Private Investment. As emphasized by Plosser (1992), capital formation is likely to be quantitatively more important for long-run growth rates than the original Solow (1956) model suggested. Hence, the crowding out of private investment in human and physical capital by government spending and taxation could have a sizable effect on the rate of economic growth. Landau (1983) and Cameron (1982) find such crowding out for physical capital formation.

Crowding Out of Private Production. Increased government demand for labor will put an upward pressure on real wages and hence crowd out private sector employment (Virén and Koskela 2000). When the government expands its activities and employs more labor, aggregate demand for labor goes up, real wages increase, and fewer jobs in the private sector will cover labor and capital costs. Private employers will respond to this by shedding labor on the margin.

Institutional Sclerosis and Rent-Seeking. Olson (1982) has suggested that organized interest groups tend to evolve, and they strive to obtain advantages for themselves in the form of legislation or transfers that have the growth-retarding side effect of worsening the functioning of the market economy. The scope for interest group action of this kind is likely to be greater in countries with larger public sectors. Similarly, in the case of a large public sector, the potential profits from rent-seeking activities are larger. This may lead to a greater diversion of resources into unproductive use, as discussed by Buchanan (1980).

Weighing the Positive against the Negative Effects

As can be seen above, we have no reason to expect a clear relationship between government size and economic growth—on the contrary. But under some circumstances, there is a pattern. The most basic tasks for government, such as protecting property rights and providing basic health care and education, can be accomplished at low or relatively low levels of taxation.

When taxes are low, distortions are also low, and there is less scope for rent-seeking simply because less money is channeled through government budgets. On the other hand, if productive government expenditure brings decreasing returns, the negative effect of taxes may at some point dominate over the positive effect of growth-promoting government activities. In fact, as pointed out by Swedish economist Jonas Agell (1996), the distortionary effect of taxation is proportional in size to the squared tax rate. This means that distortions are low for low levels of taxation, but as taxes increase, the distortions grow rapidly, and beyond a certain point they become extremely large.

For this reason, a careful reading of the existing literature suggests that the relationship between government size and growth is positive for low levels of government size and most likely negative when government is big. The question, then, is whether Western democracies have grown beyond the point where government becomes an impediment to growth. This empirical question is the focus of the next chapter.

2

What Do Existing Studies Show?

The volume of economic research on growth is huge. Luckily, there are some obvious ways of narrowing down the number of studies to manageable proportions. One is to focus mainly on relatively new studies, for at least three good reasons:

- Newer studies tend to use improved statistical techniques and make use of recent advances in computational power.

- Newer studies typically benefit from the results obtained in previous studies, taking into account what we know so far.

- Newer studies have access to longer data series, data from more countries, and data of better quality.

Some of the early studies published were actually only slightly more advanced than the scatter plots we present in chapter 1. This does not, of course, mean that all new studies are qualitatively superior to earlier ones. But average studies today are typically more informative than similar ones done in the 1980s. For this reason, we put more emphasis on the former, and focus exclusively on those published in scientific journals—that is, journals that subject papers to anonymous peer review by other scholars before accepting them for publication.

Besides focusing on newer, peer-reviewed studies, we make use of two strands of literature. Obviously, we summarize studies that focus explicitly on the relationship between government size and economic growth. But we also make use of empirical studies aiming at the more general question, what explains economic growth? Both types of literature have recently improved substantially for exactly the three reasons spelled out above.

A number of issues arise when reviewing existing research. The most important is probably the measure of government size. As discussed above, there are several possible measures to use, and different studies have used different measures.

Total government expenditure is the sum of all public expenditure (local, regional, and central) in all areas. A common mistake is to use only central government expenditure, a measure that is misleading because some countries are more decentralized than others.[1]

Expenditure can roughly be divided into public transfers (social insurance schemes and cash redistribution), public consumption (when the public sector hires people to provide certain goods and services, such as defense, health care, and education), and public investment (such as expenditure on infrastructure).

To finance public expenditure, governments collect taxes. If public budgets were always balanced, total revenue would equal total expenditure, but because they are not, this is often not the case. In practice, total tax revenue is typically lower than total expenditure, partly because governments have some nontax revenue, and partly because governments sometimes run deficits to finance their expenditure.

As with public expenditure, the federal structure of taxes varies among countries, with the bulk of the tax burden in some being at the central level, while the local level is the most important in others. Note also that the level of taxation is measured as the ratio of tax revenue to GDP, and thus says nothing about the degree of progressivity in taxes, or to what extent taxes are levied on labor, consumption, capital, and/or particular goods, such as energy or alcohol. Similarly, the ratio of total expenditure to GDP says nothing about the relative distribution of expenditure among, for example, investment, education, and social assistance.

Early Cross-Country Studies

A number of early cross-country studies, such as Cameron (1982), Landau (1983), and Marlow (1986), have found a negative relationship between government size and economic growth. These studies are summarized in table 2-1.

TABLE 2-1
SOME EARLY CROSS-COUNTRY STUDIES

Study	Measure of government size	Number of countries and time period	Effect of government size on growth
Cameron (1982)	Public consumption	48 countries, 1961–76	Negative
Landau (1983)	Public expenditure	19 countries, 1960–79	Negative
Marlow (1986)	Total expenditure, social expenditure (both levels and growth)	19 countries, 1960–80	Negative

NOTE: For example, Marlow (1986) concludes that "[a]nalysis of government expenditure data of 19 industrialized countries over the period 1960–1980 supports the view that public sector size retards overall economic growth" (152).

While seemingly convincing, the results of early studies have been criticized. Saunders (1986) summarizes the use of simple aggregate cross-country regression analysis to investigate the relationships between public sector size and economic performance. A central conclusion of his is that

> the results indicate how sensitive any conclusions are to the measure of government size selected, the time-period investigated and the countries included in the sample. Such factors, in combination with a lack of rigor in specification and evaluation of hypotheses, explain the divergency [sic!] of results produced by earlier studies adopting the cross-country framework (52).

Focusing on Marlow's 1986 study, Saunders (1988) talks in his conclusion of "the extreme sensitivity of Marlow's results to the countries included in the sample (particularly Japan), to the time period, and to the other variables included in the analysis" (284).

Some newer cross-country studies do exist. For example, Grier and Tullock (1989) study 113 countries, including 24 OECD countries, over the period 1951–80. Their measure is the growth of public consumption, which (with the exception of Asia) is negatively related to economic growth. Over a long period like this, the negative effect is highly expected. Even if we assume no growth effects from a large public sector, we would expect growth to be slower during the period when taxes must be increased to finance higher public consumption. Needless to say, this does not say anything about the effect of the level of total government size.

Newer studies have been able to probe deeper into the question. Hansson and Henrekson (1994a) examine different channels through which government size could affect growth and analyze different types of government expenditure separately. They conclude that government transfers, consumption, and total outlays have consistently negative effects, while educational expenditure has a positive effect. The reason seems to be that government expenditure decreases total factor productivity, rather than the marginal productivity of labor and capital. The level of detail in this study, however, comes at the expense of having a relatively small sample of countries: fourteen over the period 1970–87.

In a recent survey, Gordon and Wang (2004) describe the conflicting results of earlier studies, noting that Agell and others (1997), Ayal and Karras (1998), and Nelson and Singh (1998) did not find statistically significant relationships between the rate of economic growth and the size of the public sector. On the other hand, the opposite result—a significant negative correlation—was found by Knack and Keefer (1995), Barro (1997, 1998a, and 1998b), and Gwartney and others (1998). What explains these conflicting results?

Nelson and Singh (1998) look at less developed countries only, supporting the idea that government size may be good for growth in poor countries with small governments. Their study says nothing concerning the relationship in rich countries.

Barro (1997) finds a significant negative effect of government consumption, excluding spending on defense and education, on growth. Barro also addresses the problem of reverse causality by using instrumental variables. It should be noted that Barro's study uses a sample of both developed and developing countries, and government consumption (excluding defense and education) is but a subset of government expenditure. Generally, it constitutes less than half of total government spending in OECD countries. And, as previously noted, the negative effect of higher taxes is expected to be nonlinear, giving rise to steeply increased distortions beyond a certain point.

Ayal and Karras (1998) study the correlation between various components of economic freedom and the annual growth rate of GDP per capita over the period 1975–90, using a sample of 58 countries. They test the relationship between government size and economic growth only implicitly, because some measures of government size are included in the economic freedom index they use. They do find various aspects of economic freedom linked to growth when controlling for initial income, investments, and population growth. According to the authors, the primary contribution of their paper is the identification of six elements of economic freedom which are shown to be statistically significantly correlated with multifactor productivity and capital accumulation. These are low money growth rate; small role played by government enterprises; rare negative real interest rates; small difference between official and black market exchange rates; large size of the traded-goods sector; and freedom of citizens to engage in capital transactions with foreigners.

Most relevant to us is the study by Agell and others (1997), which shows that the negative bivariate correlation between government size and growth disappears when controlling for initial GDP and demography, using average annual growth and average government size (tax share and expenditure share) for OECD countries in 1970–90. While highly illustrative, this study shows little more than that conclusions based on cross-country comparisons are sensitive to the specification of the empirical model. Introducing control variables can easily change the coefficient on government size.[2]

In other words, it is possible to produce, using cross-country evidence, a seemingly convincing case that countries with bigger governments grow more slowly—the study by Gwartney and others (1998) is an example. It is also possible to question these results by including other factors in the analysis. However, although Agell and colleagues and some other scholars have been able to show that a significant negative effect of government size on economic growth can sometimes be annulled by introducing additional control variables or changing the econometric specification, obtaining significant results of the opposite sign is virtually impossible.

Rather than spending more time on early studies with conflicting results, we now turn to some more recent and advanced studies. The method described in the next section was developed to handle the problems that arise when there is uncertainty about what variables to include in the analysis.

More Sophisticated Studies A:
Bayesian Averaging of Classical Estimates (BACE)

As mentioned, one thing we learn from early cross-country studies is that results are highly sensitive to what other variables are included in the model. So how do we know what model to trust? Well, we don't. But the confusion in early cross-country studies can now partially be handled by using a method called Bayesian averaging of classical estimates. The model was developed and first used by Doppelhofer and others (2004). They noted—as we have noted above—that while several variables have been said to affect growth, many of them are significant only in some regressions.

The authors therefore constructed an algorithm that automatically ran tens of thousands of different regressions. Each regression selected a subset of variables from a set of sixty-seven factors that potentially explain economic growth. Mathematically, there are 2^{67} different possible models. Using a standard approach, any human researcher would have the time and patience to run perhaps one thousand of these, and then select a few regressions suitable for the study. Needless to say, one might expect a researcher wishing to find a negative effect of a particular variable to be more inclined to include this variable in the regression, and to show results where it had the desired sign.

The BACE algorithm handles this by requiring the researcher to supply one single parameter: the number of explanatory variables that should be included in the model. The algorithm then runs regressions and generates the average coefficient for each variable, weighted by the goodness-of-fit of each model. In other words, assuming that all sixty-seven variables are initially equally likely to be included in the model, some variables will increase their inclusion probability, and, conditional on inclusion, the BACE algorithm will give the coefficient based on a weighted average, where weights are determined by how well each possible model explains the data. To test the robustness of BACE results, it is enough to vary the model size, typically from three to seven variables.

TABLE 2-2
THIRTEEN VARIABLES THAT ROBUSTLY EXPLAIN
AVERAGE ANNUAL GROWTH IN 1960–1996

Variable	Mean	Standard deviation	Effect
Life expectancy in 1960	53.72	12.06	0.97%
Enrollment rate in primary education in 1960	73%	29%	0.78%
Population density in coastal (within 100 km of coastline) area	146.9	509.83	0.46%
Fraction of population Confucian	2%	8%	0.43%
Share of years with open economy between 1950 and 1994	36%	34%	0.42%
Fraction of population Muslim	15%	30%	0.37%
Fraction of population Buddhist	5%	17%	0.36%
Fraction of GDP in mining	5%	8%	0.30%
Government consumption as a share of GDP in 1961	12%	7%	−0.33%
Average of five different indices of ethnolinguistic fractionalization	0.35	0.30	−0.34%
Average investment price level between 1960 and 1964	92	54	−0.45%
Index of malaria prevalence in 1966	0.34	0.43	−0.68%
Initial GDP per capita (logged value)	7.35	0.9	−0.77%

SOURCE: Doppelhofer et al. 2004.
NOTE: Dummy variables for East Asia (with a positive growth effect), Africa, Latin America, and former Spanish colony (all negatively correlated with growth) are not reported. Effect is the effect in percentage points on annual growth rate from an increase by one standard deviation.

What Doppelhofer and colleagues did was to apply the BACE method to a sample of 88 countries averaged over the time period 1960–96. Among sixty-seven variables, thirteen were robust in the sense that their inclusion probability was increased when confronted with actual data. It is worth noting that among these thirteen, several were geographic dummy variables. This basically says that there is something unexplained in certain regions that systematically affects growth. Table 2-2 summarizes the findings from the BACE analysis in Doppelhofer and others (2004).

Using the same methodology and data, Jones and Schneider (2006) show that average national IQ levels also belong in the group of variables that robustly affects growth (in this case positively).

Table 2-2 should be read and interpreted as follows: Among the variables deemed robust in explaining growth, the greatest effect comes from life expectancy in 1960. The effect reports how the annual growth rate changes if the variable increases by one standard deviation.[3] Thus, countries with twelve years of higher life expectancy experienced an annual growth rate one percentage point higher, on average, in the 1960–96 period. Another large positive effect emanates from enrollment in primary education and from having more people living at or close to the coast.

Among the variables with a negative effect, the initial level of government consumption actually has the smallest effect, but it is not trivial in size: Countries with government consumption at 19 percent rather than 12 percent of GDP experienced an annual growth rate one-third of a percentage point lower as a result. On the other hand, the total government share of GDP is not included in table 2-2, because this measure of government size was significant in only 58 percent of the regressions, and its inclusion probability decreased during the BACE procedure.

The BACE study by Doppelhofer and others was pathbreaking in the way it handled the problems often encountered in earlier studies of results changing when the set of control variables was changed. But the study is far from perfect when it comes to answering questions regarding the effects of government size and growth in rich countries. Most countries in the Doppelhofer sample are low- and middle-income countries. Furthermore, relating average growth in the 1960–96 period to government size around 1960 says nothing about the consequences of the expansion of government size that took place in most countries during the period. In the next section we turn to some recent studies that focus on the evolution of growth and government size in rich countries over time.

More Sophisticated Studies B: Fixed Effects Panel Studies

Despite the recent improvements in statistical techniques used to analyze differences among countries, there is always a risk that the differences are

TABLE 2-3
RECENT PANEL DATA STUDIES

Study	Measure of government size	Number of countries and time period	Results
Fölster and Henrekson (2001)	Total tax revenue, total government expenditure	22–29 rich countries (7 rich non-OECD countries used as robustness test), 1970–95	Robust and significant negative effect from government expenditure, slightly less robust negative effect for total tax revenue.
Dar and AmirKhalkhali (2002)	Total government expenditure	19 OECD countries, 1971–99	Significant negative effect. The authors also run country-specific regressions, finding a significant negative effect in 16 out of 19 countries.
Agell et al. (2006)	Total tax revenue, total government expenditure	22–23 OECD countries	Results in Fölster and Henrekson (2001) cannot be given a causal interpretation due to simultaneity.
Romero-Avila and Strauch (2008)	Total and disaggregated revenue, total and disaggregated expenditure	15 EU countries, 1960–2001. Annual data.	Negative and significant effect for total revenue and total expenditure. Results for disaggregated revenue: negative and significant for direct taxes, insignificant for indirect taxes and social security contributions. Results for disaggregated expenditure: negative and significant effect from government consumption and transfers, significant positive effect from government investments.

NOTE: For 3 of 19 countries, Dar and AmirKhalkhali report a nonsignificant relationship: negative but insignificant in Norway and Sweden; positive but insignificant in the United States.

driven by some omitted variable. One way of handling this is to use information on changes within countries over time. When doing this, it is typically assumed that omitted variables that cause variation in growth among countries are constant within each country over time. If they are, indeed, constant over time, we do not need to know what these variables are, as their effect is being picked up by the so-called country fixed effect. The relationship among other variables of interest is then estimated using variation during the time period.

While it has some advantages, it must be noted that the fixed effects methodology eliminates the cross-sectional information in the data. Hence, any inferences must be drawn largely from time series information within countries. If only a little variation occurs in government size within countries over time, fixed effects studies may falsely indicate no negative growth effect from big government.

To do panel analysis, the variables of interest must, in fact, vary over time, and reliable data on this variation must exist. Recently, some reasonably reliable panel datasets have been used to analyze the relationship between government size and growth. Table 2-3 summarizes four such studies.

As indicated in table 2-3, there is still some controversy, but it is, in fact, of a slightly different nature. In their abstract, Fölster and Henrekson (2001, 1501) conclude:

> Our general finding is that the more the econometric problems are addressed, the more robust the relationship between government size and economic growth appears.

Their results are questioned, however, by Agell and others (2006), followed by a reply by Fölster and Henrekson (2006). The conclusion from the debate is that the correlation may be less robust when only OECD countries are included, and that causality (and not just correlation) is harder to establish using instrumental variables. The controversy is centered on regressions using first differences. As pointed out by Barro (1997), first differencing tends to emphasize measurement error over signal, and measurement error when using first differences of explanatory variables in the regression tends to bias the estimated coefficient of these variables toward zero.

These points deserve to be taken seriously. As noted in chapter 1, the OECD countries are not a random sample of rich countries. They are, in fact, united by their commitment to democracy and to a liberal market economic system, working explicitly to boost growth and living standards.[4] Thus, the fact that adding seven non-OECD countries to the analysis gives

TABLE 2-4
THE BERGH AND KARLSSON STUDY (2010)

Measure of government size	Number of countries and time period	Results
Total tax revenue, total government expenditure	24–27 OECD countries, 1970–2005	Robust and negative effects for both total tax revenue and total government expenditure

a more robust negative correlation strengthens the view that such a correlation actually exists.[5]

The second part of the criticism is that even if a correlation exists, it is harder to establish the causal effect from government size on growth, as it is possible that the causality goes the other way as well. It could be that big government is a result of low growth, rather than the other way around. In fact, this is an important point, to which we will return below. First, however, we will describe one of the most recent studies published, and so far the only one we know of that combines the advantages of the BACE method with the advantages of using panel data—namely, a 2010 study by Bergh and Karlsson.

Combining BACE with Panel Data

Bergh and Karlsson (2010) adapt the BACE method to panel data and apply it to the same dataset used by Fölster and Henrekson (2001). They also update the dataset, adding ten years of observations, and run the algorithm both on the original data for the period 1970–95 and the updated dataset covering the 1970–2005 period. The study and its results are summarized in table 2-4.

Four variables were deemed robust in both the 1970–95 and the 1970–2005 datasets: government size, relative GDP level, inflation, and savings (all negatively correlated with growth, except for savings). Table 2-5 compares the magnitudes of these effects by showing how much annual growth

TABLE 2-5

THE GROWTH EFFECTS OF FOUR VARIABLES FOUND ROBUST

Variable	Mean	Standard deviation	Effect
Tax revenue, share of GDP	33.6%	9%	–0.9%
Initial per-capita income relative to the OECD average	1	0.29	–2%
Inflation	0.08	0.016	–2.7%
Gross national saving, share of GDP	0.24	0.08	0.2%

SOURCE: Bergh and Karlsson (2010).
NOTE: Effect measures the estimated growth effect in percentage points of an increase of one standard deviation in the variable in question.

would change if the variable were to increase by one standard deviation. We see that inflation varies substantially among the countries in the sample, and also that inflation seems to be really bad for growth. We also see that the relative position of a country is important: Those that are richer than the OECD average grow more slowly, and those that are poorer grow more rapidly.

More interestingly, tax revenue as a share of GDP is one of the four variables singled out by the BACE procedure. A tax revenue one standard deviation higher is associated with annual growth nine-tenths of a percentage point lower. This is a relatively large effect in comparison with previous studies. Finally, it should be noted that when Bergh and Karlsson apply the BACE method to the longer time period, 1970–2005, including the most recent data, government expenditure as a share of GDP is also robustly negatively related to growth.

To conclude, the studies by Fölster and Henrekson (2001), Dar and AmirKhalkhali (2002), Romero-Avila and Strauch (2008), and Bergh and Karlsson (2010) in our view basically settle the issue: *In rich countries, there is, indeed, a robust negative correlation between total government size and growth.* Table 2-6 summarizes the size of the effect according to the studies we consider to be the best. As can be seen, for both taxes and expenditure, coefficients vary from –0.05 to –0.1, which means that an increase of ten percentage points in tax revenue as a share of GDP is associated with annual growth between one-half and one percentage point lower.

TABLE 2-6

COMPARISON OF ESTIMATES IN DIFFERENT STUDIES—DEPENDENT
VARIABLE: ANNUAL GROWTH RATE OF REAL GDP PER CAPITA

Study	Coefficient on total tax revenue (share of GDP)	Coefficient on total public expenditure (share of GDP)
Bergh and Karlsson (2010) (BACE, OECD, 1970–95)	–0.11	Not robust
Bergh and Karlsson (2010) (BACE, OECD, 1970–2005)	–0.10	–0.09
Fölster and Henrekson (2001), table 2. (Fixed effects panel, OECD, 1970–95)	–0.05 (not significant)	–0.07 (significant at 5%)
Romero-Avila and Strauch (2008), table 5. (Fixed effects panel, EU15, 1960–2001)	–0.06 to –0.07 (significant at 5% or 1%)	–0.05 (significant at 1%)
Dar and AmirKhalkhali (2002), table 3. (Random effects panel, 19 OECD countries, 1971–99)	n.a.	Significant negative effects in 16 out of 19 countries: from –0.05 in Finland and Belgium to –0.16 in Portugal.

NOTE: For 3 out of 19 countries in this study, Dar and AmirKhalkhali report a nonsignificant relationship: negative but insignificant in Norway and Sweden, positive but insignificant in the United States.

So far, however, we have not settled the issue of causality—that is, what causes what? In the next section we discuss this issue further.

Is the Negative Correlation Due to Reverse Causality?

As we have seen, there seems to be a fairly robust negative correlation between government size and economic growth. But correlation does not imply causality. What if there are mechanisms that imply that countries with slower growth have larger governments? If so, slow growth causes big government, and not the other way around. This is known as the problem of reverse causality.

In the early cross-country studies, the problem of reverse causality is typically handled by including explanatory variables that predate the variable to be explained—in this case, economic growth. The reasoning in, for example, the BACE analysis by Doppelhofer and others (2004) is that the average annual growth rate from 1960 to 1996 can hardly explain the situation causally in 1960. It seems more likely, therefore, that the size of public consumption in 1960 causes lower growth rates in subsequent years than that the average rate of growth after 1960 affects the extent of government consumption in 1960.

While the latter assertion seems reasonable enough, the use of initial values as regressors is not wholly unproblematic. It is probably hard to argue that slower growth in the 1980s and the 1990s was caused by government size as far back as in the year 1960—especially when considering that the extent of government consumption changes substantially over time.

As described above, panel studies solve this problem by using changes in government size (and other variables) within countries over time to estimate growth effects. But then the possibility of reverse causality creeps back in: From year to year, it is obvious that, to some extent, government expenditure will depend on growth, and not only the other way around. The reason for this is the fact that most rich countries have some type of welfare arrangements that cause expenditure to rise when the business cycle goes down.

For example, total public expenditure peaked at the extremely high level of approximately 70 percent of GDP in Sweden in 1993. This resulted from very high expenditure on unemployment benefits, which were, in turn, caused by high layoffs. In general, social expenditure provides stabilizers that automatically underbalance the government budget in times of economic downturns. On the other hand, in boom years, when growth rates are higher, fewer people will be unemployed, and public expenditure shares will be lower. For this reason, a negative correlation between public expenditure and economic growth is to be expected in the short run, and finding a negative correlation is, therefore, no proof that high expenditure causes low growth.

For taxes, the same reasoning means that we risk finding no link even if there is a causal link from taxes to growth. This is so for several reasons.

First of all, most countries have at least slightly progressive tax schemes. This means that when growth increases, so will tax revenue, and the ratio of tax revenue to GDP will increase. Another reason is that the taxation of capital gains and profits results in higher revenue when the economy is booming. Both effects mean that, in the data, high taxes will correlate positively with rapid growth, but causality runs from growth to tax revenue, not the other way around.

The upshot of these important mechanisms is that a negative coefficient on government expenditure in growth regressions need not imply that big government causes slower growth. On the other hand, a negative coefficient on taxes actually provides rather strong evidence that high taxes cause lower growth, because reverse causality leads us to expect a positive correlation. Bergh and Karlsson (2010) discuss this issue at some length and note that taxes are actually more robust than expenditure in their analysis, which is a strong indication that the negative relationship they find is not driven by reverse causality.

Another solution to the problem is to include a measure of business cycle variations, such as the level of unemployment or capacity utilization. A third possibility is to adjust data to filter out short-term cyclical variations.

Fölster and Henrekson (2001) use five-year averages in almost all regressions and also try the other methods in at least one of their regressions. They argue that the negative effect is robust. Romero-Avila and Strauch (2008) use annual data, but they test the robustness by using cyclically adjusted data and find that the negative effect remains.

Another way of handling the problem of reverse causality is to use so-called instrumental variables. In this case, the task is to find some variable or variables that are correlated with government size but not with economic growth, and use the variation in these variables to predict government size. Then, a second-stage regression examines whether these predicted values have a negative effect on growth. It should be noted that both Fölster and Henrekson (2001) and Romero-Avila and Strauch (2008) do test their results using instrumental variable estimation and find robustness—but the lack of good instruments for government size means that the issue has not yet been completely settled.[6] This problem plagues many econometric studies of important phenomena, preventing researchers from giving causal interpretations even to strong correlations.

Results from Other Research Explaining Growth

Several studies that focus on studying the relationship between something else and growth can also tell us about government size because they control for it. In these studies, government size is usually measured by government consumption as a share of GDP, and most studies find a negative and significant effect.

Examples include Yang (2008), who studies the relationship between foreign direct investment and growth for 110 countries in the 1973–2002 period. When controlling for black market premium (significant negative effect), financial development (ambiguous effect), and openness (significant positive effect), a negative growth effect of public consumption is found.

Loayza and Ranciere (2006) study the relationship between financial development and growth, using data from 75 countries during the period 1960–2000. Again, government consumption as a share of GDP is strongly negatively related to growth.

Bekaert and others (2005) study 95 countries during the 1980–1997 period. They find a negative but insignificant effect of government consumption on growth. Control variables include black market premium, legal origin, efficiency of the judicial system, quality of institutions, corruption, and bureaucratic quality.

Ehrlich and Francis (1999) study the relationship between bureaucratic corruption and endogenous economic growth, looking at a panel of 152 countries during the period 1960–92. Total government spending as a share of GDP is often—but not always—negatively related to growth.

Concluding Remarks

In our view, the best studies published so far are the one by Romero-Avila and Strauch (2008) and that by Bergh and Karlsson (2010). The periods studied are long, the countries are highly similar, data quality is high, and the authors check the robustness of their results in several ways. Romero-Avila and Strauch also examine the effects of different types of taxes and expenditure and check their results for reverse causality. It is no surprise that both these studies are the most recently published ones that we have reviewed, as the quality of studies is continually improving.

Even if there is consensus that growth and government size are negatively related in rich countries, some countries, such as the Scandinavian welfare states, exhibit relatively high growth despite having large governments. Apparently, we must account for other factors that influence growth. In the next chapter, we describe one of the most recent advances in the growth literature: the importance of institutional quality.

3

The Growth Effects of
Institutional Quality

The most recent trend in research on economic growth is to investigate the role of institutions. Following works like North (1987), several studies have tested, and found strong support for, the idea that certain fundamental institutional arrangements are crucial for economic growth. The rule of law and well-functioning property rights are probably the most important in this respect. In a famous paper, Rodrik and others (2004) claim that certain types of institutional quality—especially property rights—are more important for growth than such factors as geography and trade.

Several literature reviews have recently confirmed the consensus that institutions matter for growth. Abdiweli (2003) has surveyed existing evidence, and his own research confirms that judicial efficiency, low levels of corruption, a well-organized public bureaucracy, and well-defined private property rights covary positively with high levels of growth. The risk of breach of contract and risk of government expropriation have clear negative effects on growth, according to Abdiweli. In another important survey, Doucouliagos and Ulubasoglu (2006) review and evaluate fifty-two other studies that examine the link between economic freedom (measured in several different ways) and growth. They conclude that economic freedom "has a robust positive effect on economic growth regardless of how it is measured" (68). Berggren and Jordahl (2005) compare different types of economic freedom, and find that security of property rights and the integrity of the legal system are the ones most robustly related to growth.

The relationship between the concepts of "institutional quality" and "economic freedom" in the literature is not entirely clear. Institutional quality is the broader of the two, not clearly defined simply because we do not know exactly what types of institutions are beneficial. On the other hand, economic freedom typically refers to the Economic Freedom Index of the Fraser Institute, a commonly used index that quantifies certain aspects of economic freedom. As Gwartney and others (2004) point out, the Economic Freedom Index measures both longer-term institutional variables, such as the quality of the legal system, and shorter-term public policies, such as marginal tax rates; but the term "institutional quality" is often used to refer to both.

Whether levels of institutional quality or changes (that is, reforms) matter more for growth is a source of disagreement. In two similar papers, De Haan and Sturm (2000) and Sturm and De Haan (2001) conduct a series of thorough analyses of the relationship between economic freedom and growth. Applying the method of extreme bounds analysis,[1] their overall finding is that the level of economic freedom is not robustly related to economic growth, but that changes in economic freedom have a robust impact on economic growth. On the other hand, Dawson (2003) uses so-called Granger tests to assess the relationship and finds that the level of economic freedom, especially the level of property rights, is an important cause of economic growth. So far, no consensus has emerged.

Why Do Institutions Matter?

The reasons institutions matter for growth are actually quite intuitive and easy to understand. An individual who is in a position to work, trade, or innovate wants to know that such efforts will be rewarding. He or she will want to know which rules concern contracts and agreements, profits, and wages. If information is insufficient, numerous investments and work efforts become too risky to undertake. For the same reason, it is important to be certain about the value of money in the future; whenever uncertainty prevails, lenders will demand a higher interest rate, and many potential investment projects are rendered unprofitable.

The fundament for prosperity in a market economy is the voluntary exchange of goods and services, as well as the free exchange of ideas and knowledge. As discussed in chapter 1, the most basic theoretical reason for expecting a negative effect of taxes on economic development is that transactions that would take place without taxation may not take place when buyers or sellers must pay taxes on top of the price on which they agreed. Taxation introduces a wedge between the buyer's and seller's valuations of the transaction, and as a result many transactions are no longer mutually beneficial and do not take place.

The price for a good or a service (with or without taxes) is, however, only one part of the total cost of a transaction. Other costs include, for example, those for buyers and sellers to find each other, to reach an agreement and mutually and credibly assure each other that they will, in fact, adhere to it, and possibly also to agree on how to settle potential disputes. Well-defined property rights, a well-functioning legal system, and a stable currency are factors that lower transaction costs drastically.

The role of institutions can also explain a regularity known as the resource curse: the fact that many poor countries are poor despite having valuable natural resources. In the absence of good institutions, these resources are the source of conflicts, corruption, and detrimental behaviors that obstruct growth. Higher institutional quality brings both laws and social norms that ease conflict resolution and lower transaction costs, fostering economic development.[2]

De Soto (2000) sheds light on how the absence of effective property rights can explain the lack of economic growth in the world's poorest countries. When houses cannot be mortgaged because they were built without permits and titles, investments fail to materialize. Ambiguous property rights cause resources to be put into the handling of conflicts instead of into prosperity-enhancing production.

A concept somewhat related to economic freedom is globalization, a term usually used to describe the increased movement of goods, people, and capital across national borders. Without doubt, "globalization" is something of a buzzword, and some popular accounts of the phenomenon have been criticized for being both vague and only partially true, as argued, for example, by Leamer in his 2007 review of Thomas Friedman's best-selling book *The World Is Flat*. Nevertheless, globalization can be given a precise meaning. A new index by Dreher (2006) divides it into economic, social, and political globalization, respectively, and quantifies these three aspects according to several measurable indicators. Most important, Dreher shows that this globalization index, known as the KOF Index, is positively related to economic growth.

Thus, any discussion of economic growth must take institutional factors such as economic freedom and globalization into account. As will become clear below, this is especially important in the debate regarding the effect of government size on growth.

The Surprising Correlation between Big Government and Reforms Furthering Economic Freedom

As mentioned above, globalization can be measured using the KOF Index developed by Dreher (2006). Several options are available to measure economic freedom, but the Economic Freedom Index developed by the Fraser Institute is still one of the most commonly used in economic research. This index consists of five dimensions: size of government, legal structure and security of property rights, access to sound money, freedom to exchange with foreigners, and regulation of credit, labor, and business. Using several indicators in each, the five dimensions are weighed together in a composite index, where 0 indicates the lowest and 10 the highest degree of economic freedom.

Using these indices, a somewhat surprising fact emerges: Countries with larger government sectors have, on average, had greater increases in economic freedom and globalization between 1970 and 2000. In figure 3-1, we illustrate the increase in index values for economic freedom and globalization for countries with different sizes of government.[3]

The scatter plots show that countries that had big governments in the 1970s increased their degrees of globalization and economic freedom more than other countries—and they still had big governments in 2000.

To some extent, the pattern can be explained by the simple fact that countries with big governments were typically those that had below-average economic freedom and globalization to begin with. As demonstrated by Bergh (2006), the pattern today is the opposite of that in 1970, with the Scandinavian welfare states having more economic freedom and being more globalized than countries in continental Europe.

As expected, the Scandinavian countries have during the entire period low economic freedom in the first dimension, related to government size. But in the 1970–2000 period, the Scandinavian welfare states (Sweden,

FIGURE 3-1

INCREASE FROM 1970 TO 2000 IN KOF INDEX VALUES
OF GLOBALIZATION AND ECONOMIC FREEDOM INDEX (EFI)
COMPARED TO TAX SHARE OF GDP IN 1970

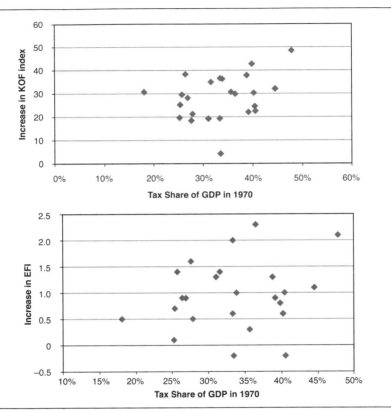

SOURCE: Authors' calculations based on data in Bergh and Karlsson (2010).

Finland, Norway, and Denmark) increased their average level of economic freedom in the four remaining dimensions more than the southwestern European welfare states and more than liberal welfare states.[4] This means they improved their legal structure and security of property rights, access to sound money, and freedom to trade internationally, and decreased their regulation of credit, labor, and business.

The different patterns in the evolution of economic freedom in other countries are important, because the studies referred to in the previous section do not take these institutional reforms into account—a failure that causes an omitted-variable problem in them. The studies by Romero-Avila and Strauch (2008), Agell and others (2006), and Fölster and Henrekson (2001) cover more or less the entire time period during which these reforms took place without accounting for institutional development.

Especially if De Haan and Sturm (2000) are correct in their contention that changes in economic freedom promote growth, this means that, for example, economic growth in the Scandinavian welfare states has been higher thanks to institutional reforms during the 1980s and 1990s. If Dawson (2003) is correct in that the level (rather than increases) of economic freedom is a cause of growth, the high level attained by the Scandinavian welfare states by the mid-1990s most likely contributed to the relatively high level of growth recently attained in these countries.

Theoretically, there are actually a number of reasons economic freedom and globalization may be especially important for countries with big governments. Due to trends like increasing mobility of the tax base, globalization has often been depicted as a potential threat to the welfare state.[5] There was talk of a "race to the bottom," in which the forces of globalization would put pressure on welfare states to lower taxes and welfare benefits.[6] Today, however, the consensus is that welfare states have survived (although a bit trimmed), and no race to the bottom has occurred.[7]

This is less surprising than it may seem. Often overlooked have been several mechanisms through which both globalization and economic freedom may positively affect the welfare state. Economic openness and free trade create more opportunities for increased division of labor. With openness comes access not only to new products but also to knowledge, technologies, and larger markets. In line with these arguments, Iversen (2005) has proposed that extensive welfare states are likely to run into problems unless they apply a policy of economic openness:

> Labor-intensive, low-productivity jobs do not thrive in the context of high social protection and intensive labor-market regulation, and without international trade countries cannot specialize in high value-added services. Lack of international trade and competition, therefore, not the growth of these, is the cause of current employment problems in high-protection countries (74).

According to this view, the negative effects of extensive transfers, high tax wedges, and stringent labor market regulations can, at least to some extent, be offset by economic openness, because openness allows welfare states to specialize in high-value-added services. More research is needed, but some support for this idea is found in the study by Bergh and Karlsson (2010), where exports and freedom to trade are found to promote growth.

Conclusion: Not Only Size Matters

Many studies suggest that total tax revenue matters for growth, but how taxes are designed also matters. Remember that Romero-Avila and Strauch (2008) find a significant negative effect from direct income taxes, but do not find a significant effect for indirect taxes and social security contributions. Similarly, Widmalm (2001) finds that taxes on personal income as a share of total tax revenue impede growth. She finds a similar effect for tax progressivity. And, as already noted, according to standard microeconomic theory, tax distortions are proportional to the square of the tax rate.[8]

In other words, research suggests that, for a given level of total taxation, a country can reduce the negative consequences for the economy by collecting taxes in a smarter way. This means, for example, reducing the progressivity of the tax system. And this is exactly what most countries have done, including those with very high levels of average taxation. As shown by Curzon Price (2008), the trend toward lower top marginal tax rates is unambiguous in almost all countries. But lower tax rates have—generally—not been associated with lower tax revenue or smaller government. Rather, Curzon Price argues, institutional competition has forced countries to introduce less distortionary tax systems.[9]

The idea that countries with high taxation have learned to extract tax revenue more efficiently is consistent with a finding by Dar and AmirKhalkhali (2002), who show that size of government had a statistically significant negative impact on total factor productivity growth during the 1970s and 1980s—but not during the 1990s. Similarly, Romero-Avila and Strauch (2008) find that different types of expenditure have different growth effects. Public consumption often impedes growth, while public investments may well enhance it.

In reality, it is still true that in countries with very high aggregate taxes as a share of GDP, it is virtually impossible to avoid high rates of taxation of labor. This is particularly so if increased economic and financial integration puts downward pressure on capital taxes. As we will explain in the next chapter, high rates of labor taxation make it unprofitable to produce many personal services in the formal economy, since competition from the untaxed "do-it-yourself" and black market sectors goes up when labor taxes are increased. In the standard neoclassical growth model, this only affects the level of income and not its growth rate. But when services are provided by professionals, incentives emerge to invest in new knowledge, to develop more effective tools, to develop superior contractual arrangements, and to create more flexible organizational structures. Thus, higher rates of personal taxation reduce the scope for entrepreneurial expansion into new market activities that economize on time use or that supply close substitutes for home-produced services. And without the emergence of new service jobs replacing traditional manufacturing jobs, the demand for tax-financed transfers will increase. This puts an upward pressure on the tax and expenditure ratios, which provides an additional channel resulting in lower economic growth.

4

Deficient Marketization of Household Production in High-Tax Societies

While the neoclassical model focused on the contribution of conventional measures of labor and physical capital as the basic reproducible inputs, early implementations of it recognized the existence of a large, unexplained residual, which was generally ascribed to the unaccounted role of technology.[1] The quality of the labor input, as measured by education, skill, and entrepreneurship, was an obvious missing link in this accounting experiment. This may have set the stage for turning attention to investment in human beings. An important paper by Robert Lucas (1988) on the mechanics of economic growth ascribed persistent, long-term growth in per-capita income and consumption to continuous investments in human capital. The model replaced the neoclassical model's reliance on exogenous shifts in "technology" with endogenous optimal investment in human capital. But for investment in increasingly specialized knowledge to be profitable, the division of labor needs to increase continuously, and the use of this knowledge needs to be intense, because investment costs are independent of the intensity with which acquired skills are employed.

A large share of all work, most notably household work, is performed outside the market. Cross-country comparisons of industry-level employment also point to considerable scope for substitution of certain economic activities between the market and nonmarket sectors.[2] In Sweden, studies indicate that in the early 1990s more time was spent on household production than market production.[3] Furthermore, paid work not reported to the tax authorities was estimated to be approximately 10 percent of the hours worked in the marketplace. In a detailed industry-level comparison of Sweden and the United States, Davis and Henrekson (2005) demonstrate

TABLE 4-1

PAID WORK, UNPAID WORK, AND TIME WITH CHILDREN IN SWEDEN AND
THE UNITED STATES, LATEST AVAILABLE YEAR FROM TIME-USE STUDIES

Hours per year, ages 20–74	Paid work	Unpaid work	Time with children
Women			
Sweden	1,050	1,180	180
United States	1,230	1,120	250
Men			
Sweden	1,530	810	100
United States	1,810	660	105

SOURCES: *OECD in Figures 2007* (data for 2006); OECD Labor Market Database, AUTS 2005; and Eurostat Standardized Time Use Survey. For further details, see Sanandaji and Wallen (2009).
NOTE: The latest available year is 2001 for Sweden and 2005 for the United States.

that relative employment in the United States was considerably greater in household-related services, such as repair of durable goods, hotel and restaurant services, retail sales, and laundry and household work.

Marked differences also appeared between Swedish and U.S. men. U.S. men worked more in the market, while Swedish men performed substantially more household work. In particular, Swedish men were the clear international leaders in home improvement time, averaging 4 hours per week, compared to 2.8 hours for U.S. men and less than 1 hour for Japanese men. Total work time for Swedish and U.S. men was virtually identical (57.9 versus 57.8 hours). The amount of leisure time was approximately 3 hours longer per week in the United States compared to Sweden for both men and women. Thus, "Swedish men, compared to U.S. men, have less market work time, more home production time, and less leisure time."[4]

The most recent Sweden–U.S. time-use data are reported in table 4-1. Here it is also clear that both Swedish men and women work less in the market and more in the household than their U.S. counterparts.

Why is this? A strong case can be made that taxes in Sweden act as disincentives for market work and hamper the development of an extensive service sector.

FIGURE 4-1

**AVERAGE HOURS WORKED PER PERSON 15–64 YEARS OF AGE,
SWEDEN AND THE UNITED STATES, 1956–2003**

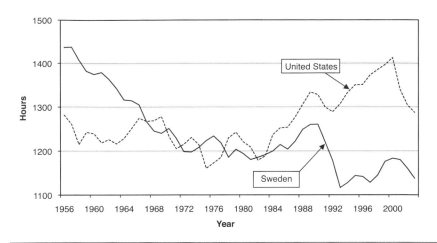

SOURCE: Rogerson (2006), as compiled from OECD sources and the Groningen Growth and Development Center.

In a well-functioning, decentralized market economy, entrepreneurs can be expected to detect and act upon the potential for starting new operations or expanding existing ones, thereby creating job opportunities. Figure 4-1 shows average work hours per person of working age from 1956 to 2003 in Sweden and the United States, respectively. Average work time has evolved along remarkably different paths in the two countries, with Americans working much less than Swedes in the 1950s and much more by the 1990s. Among Swedes ages fifteen to sixty-four, work time fell by more than 200 hours per year from 1956 to 1972. It then fluctuated in a narrow band for fifteen years, before recovering somewhat in the late 1980s and plummeting to new lows in the 1990s. Hours per working-age Swede dropped by 11.5 percent, from 1,261 in 1990 to 1,116 in 1993. In contrast, average hours among working-age Americans rose rapidly, from 1,179 in 1982 to 1,413 in 2000, and then fell sharply after 2000 from a very high base. According to these data, Americans spent 150 hours more per year in market work activity than Swedes as of 2003.

U.S. trends in recent decades indicate that the bulk of new jobs net are created through the rapid growth of an increasingly differentiated service sector. Sweden is different, because personal taxes increase the prices of goods and services. For many goods—for example, high-tech products like computers—a high price may cause the consumer to forgo a purchase or to buy a lower-quality version of the good. But with services, high labor taxes often induce consumers to produce the service themselves.[5] High rates of taxation of labor tend to make it more profitable to shift a large share of the service production to the informal economy, in particular into the "do-it-yourself" sector. Where the cost of the service consists of labor cost only, it can be shown that market production is profitable only if the following holds: [6]

$$\frac{\text{Buyer's hourly wage before tax}}{\text{Seller's hourly wage before tax}} \cdot \frac{\text{Seller's productivity}}{\text{"Do-it-yourself" productivity}} >$$

$$> \frac{(1 + \text{the VAT rate})(\ 1 + \text{social security rate})}{1 - \text{buyer's marginal tax rate}}$$

Let us call the right-hand side of this expression the tax factor.[7] The expression describes a fundamental economic relationship, which, given wage and productivity differentials, is a crucial determinant of the demarcation line between taxed and untaxed work. Low rates of taxation on labor require smaller wage differentials before tax and/or productivity differences to avoid the crowding out of professional work by unpaid work in cases where unpaid (or black market) work is feasible.

In the early 2000s, the tax factor in Sweden was in the interval 2.7–4.0, while in the United States the tax factor was generally in the 1.4–1.9 interval. Comparisons between Sweden and the United States (represented by California) show that for a professional service producer to be competitive vis-à-vis unpaid household production, the professional must have a productivity edge of 170–300 percent in Sweden, whereas 40–90 percent is sufficient in the United States in the case of equal market wage. Alternatively, in the case of equal productivity (for example, child care), the hourly wage of the buyer must exceed that of the seller by a factor of 2.7–4.0 in Sweden, whereas a factor of 1.4–1.9 is sufficient in the United States.

As a result, the emergence of a large, efficient service sector competing successfully with unpaid work is less likely in a large welfare state than in a country with lower rates of labor taxation (and higher wage dispersion). Put simply, higher rates of personal taxation discourage the market provision of goods and services that substitute closely for home-produced services. As a consequence, higher rates of personal taxation reduce the scope for entrepreneurial expansion into new market activities that economize on time use or that supply close substitutes for home-produced services.

These factors also help explain why the increased participation rate of women in the U.S. labor market in the 1960s paved the way for comprehensive marketization of household services to a greater extent than in Sweden, despite the more rapid increase in female participation rates in Sweden. The average number of hours worked by U.S. women of working age increased by 40 percent between 1975 and 1994. Measured as the average number of hours worked per working-age woman, female employment in the United States reached the level in Sweden already in the 1970s (Jonung and Persson 1993). This process occurred despite the massive expansion in public sector employment in Sweden, which increased the demand for female employment as the expansion involved predominantly "female" occupations. Furthermore, the increased public sector employment involved greater subsidies for child and elder care, work traditionally performed predominantly by women in the home.

From a static standpoint, we have seen how Sweden's tax structure frequently gets in the way of profitable transactions in the market, since high taxes lead to an inefficient allocation of labor time across tasks. In addition to these static effects, at least three distinct *dynamic* effects are likely to have an impact on long-run growth and welfare. First, less specialization in the labor force lowers productivity, because there will be less learning-by-doing. Second, less scope for specialization among workers will lower incentives to invest in specialized human capital. This follows from the fact that the return to investment in a specific skill increases in its subsequent utilization, because investment costs are independent of the intensity with which acquired skills are employed (Rosen 1983). Third, and analogous to the previous effect, the incentives to innovate are obviously weaker when specialization is lower, since a (product or process) innovation yields a smaller return the less of one's total labor time is devoted to the activity where the innovation is carried out.

The high taxation on labor would appear to frustrate seriously the evolution of a modern service-oriented economy. Thus, Sweden's high rate of taxation on labor has deprived the country of one of the most effective engines for income and wealth creation: an increasingly sophisticated division of labor and specialization. In the words of Adam Smith, "It is the great multiplication of the productions of all the different arts, in consequence of the division of labor, which occasions, in a well-governed society, that universal opulence which extends itself to the lowest ranks of the people" (1776 [1965], 11). Smith emphasized the key role of the extent of the market in limiting a further division of labor. Another, equal impediment may well be high rates of personal taxation that reduce the extent to which it is profitable for workers to make intensive use of highly specialized knowledge (Becker and Murphy 1992).

No doubt, lifestyles that involve two income earners in married or cohabiting households increase the potential demand for many household-related services.[8] If, however, the tax code to a large extent hinders the development of a modern service-oriented economy, the demands for shorter working hours and work sharing in Sweden and other European countries are easily understood. Furthermore, given Sweden's high marginal tax rate, including the effect of income-based subsidies, a reduction of working hours does not normally translate into a significant decline in income. From the perspective of the individual Swede who faces a high marginal tax rate, a reduction in working hours appears highly attractive.

Thus, high tax rates on labor frequently get in the way of socially desirable market transactions, which shift the level of income and production downward. What may be more important from a dynamic perspective is that an economy with high labor taxes is slower to adjust and provide a variety of new services in an efficient manner. This is easier to understand if we bear in mind that when services are provided by professionals, new incentives emerge to invest in new knowledge, to develop more effective tools, to develop superior contractual arrangements, to create more flexible organizational structures, and so forth. There is reason, then, to believe that the growth of service productivity will be more rapid when in the hands of a professional than when an individual chooses to produce the service him- or herself. We should, therefore, expect this mechanism to affect the growth rate and not just the level of income. Another, quite distinct, issue is the effect of taxes on the supply of entrepreneurial energy and the willingness to bear risk.[9]

This perspective helps explain two seemingly incongruous aspects of the U.S. economy compared to that of other wealthy countries. First, the United States has a relatively large fraction of employment in cleaning services, restaurants, beauty parlors, home repair, and other "old-fashioned" personal services that substitute closely for home-produced services. Second, the United States has been, and remains, the leading developer of innovative business models for the provision of time-saving services. Convenience stores, fast-food restaurants, large shopping malls, and superstores like Wal-Mart originated in the United States. More recently, Internet companies like Amazon.com, Ebay, HomeGrocer, and PeaPod are transforming shopping and distribution in important sectors of the U.S. economy.

The tax perspective explains both sets of facts as being a consequence of relatively low personal tax rates in the United States. The tax perspective also suggests that the United States is likely to continue as the leading developer of innovative business models along these lines, partly because of comparatively low personal tax rates. By the same logic, high personal tax rates constrain the scope for entrepreneurial expansion into these new market activities in other wealthy countries and, to a lesser extent, in the United States.

Conclusions and Policy Implications

Simply put, the debate about growth and government size is about the trade-off between the size of a cake and its distribution. Expanding government to split a cake differently may prove unwise if it means that the cake to be divided will grow more slowly. The late Arthur M. Okun put it brilliantly in the title of his classic 1975 book, *Equality and Efficiency: The Big Tradeoff*.

Some scholars have argued that no such tradeoff exists. For example, Lindert (2004) and Madrick (2009) have put forward arguments suggesting that the welfare state is "a free lunch" (the title of a Lindert working paper from 2003), and that research supports a "case for big government" (the title of Madrick's 2009 book). We have shown that these conclusions are clearly premature. A negative correlation between various measures of government size and economic growth in rich countries is the most frequent result presented in the recent literature.

Although increases in the economic standard of living do not necessarily translate one-to-one into increased social welfare, the correspondence is close enough to make economic growth an important policy priority. Yet clearly, for a number of reasons, a fairly large government sector relative to GDP is needed in today's wealthiest countries. The government is, in practice, the only agent that can uphold private property rights and the rule of law, provide collective goods such as national defense and basic infrastructure, and deal with positive and negative externalities.

Tanzi and Schuknecht (1997) deem that a level of public spending somewhere between 30 and 40 percent of GDP is sufficient. Countries with spending beyond this level do seem to have lower income inequality, but they do not score higher on social indicators such as life expectancy or infant mortality. Nevertheless, government spending in many OECD countries is closer to 50 percent of GDP.

There are a number of reasons to expect this additional government spending to hamper the functioning of the economic system, thereby giving rise to both static level effects and dynamic growth effects. The most important is the distortionary effect of taxation, but there is also the fact that, arguably, more efficient private production and investment are likely to be crowded out, and the scope for unproductive rent-seeking is likely to increase. Still, assessing whether these growth effects are of sizable economic significance is an empirical matter.

Our extensive review of several generations of studies exploring the relationship between the relative size of government and the rate of growth shows that a statistically negative effect is found in the majority of them. But how large is this effect? Is it large enough to be economically significant?

Policy Implications in General

With few exceptions, recent studies published in scientific journals tend to find a negative relationship between government size and economic growth in rich countries. This means that, all else equal, larger government is associated on average with significantly lower rates of growth.

Countries tend to cluster to institutions that go well together. As stressed by many observers (Freeman, for example, in a 1995 study), the Swedish welfare state can be seen as an economic model, or system, defined by a particular mixture of institutions. The mixture of institutions and the interactions among them are key determinants of economic performance. For instance, the combination of high marginal tax rates and a narrow pre-tax wage dispersion is likely to discourage labor supply under the Swedish model, but this effect is mitigated by mechanisms that restrict access to highly subsidized services to unemployed persons (Lindbeck 1982).

Moreover, around 1990, radical tax reforms were instituted in Sweden and many other high-tax countries. These reforms substantially lowered the distortionary effect of the tax system at any given level of aggregate taxation (Agell 1996). As explained in chapter 4, however, high rates of personal taxation make it very difficult to develop a large and differentiated sector for personal services, since high personal taxes in the formal sector favor unpaid household production and black market activity. To some extent

FIGURE C-1

ECONOMIC FREEDOM IN SWEDEN AND THE UNITED STATES, 1970–2006

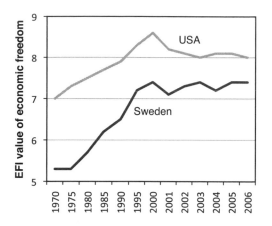

SOURCE: Gwartney et al. (2008).

this can be counteracted by strong work incentives in all transfer programs, efficient labor market programs, and some sort of earned income tax credit (EITC) that gives strong incentives for labor market participation even for low productivity workers.[1]

For this reason, high taxes may do relatively less harm in the Scandinavian countries than in the United States—but it is still not advisable for the United States to increase taxes and spending to Scandinavian levels. Moreover, since high rates of personal taxation depress market work activity, the number of hours worked per capita in the formal sector goes down, which tends both to erode the tax base and increase the demand for transfer payments. Both effects put upward pressure on the tax ratio and thereby have a negative effect on economic growth.

Institutions characterized by high levels of economic freedom are strongly linked to growth, according to recent research. The recent favorable economic performance of many high-tax countries most likely emanates from institutional reforms, which offset the negative effects of big government. The development of economic freedom is measured by the often used index of the Fraser Institute, as shown in figure C-1.

Since 1970, the difference between Sweden and the United States has decreased. Sweden has increased its index value by 40 percent, compared to 14 percent for the United States. In 2000, only Hong Kong had higher economic freedom than the United States. The conclusion is simple but important: For Sweden in the 1980s and the 1990s, it was possible to promote growth by reforming institutions toward higher degrees of economic freedom. In the United States, this option was not available because the level of economic freedom there was already very high.

Should Government Be Allowed to Grow in the United States?

It must always be remembered that the results reported in studies of the relationship between government size and growth are averages. In practice, countries with fairly efficient and noncorrupt public bureaucracies can afford to let government grow larger without experiencing a large negative growth effect. In combination with a great deal of freedom in terms of deregulated product and capital markets and welfare policies aimed at improving the functioning of the labor market, a large public sector may not be so inimical to economic growth. It will still be difficult, however, to avoid the problem discussed in chapter 4—that is, that countries with high rates of personal taxation will have trouble developing a vibrant personal service sector. This problem is likely to become increasingly important in the Scandinavian welfare states as well as in many countries in continental Europe in the future. And without the emergence of new service jobs replacing traditional manufacturing jobs, the demand for tax-financed transfers will increase. This will put an upward pressure on the tax and expenditure ratios, thereby providing an additional channel through which economic growth may be hampered.

Despite what we have said about the ability of the Scandinavian countries to combine large governments with high rates of growth in recent years, our analysis provides no case for arguing that the United States could increase the size of its government sector significantly without having to pay a fairly high price in terms of forgone economic growth. The United States is much more diverse than Scandinavia in ethnicity, level of education, competencies, and social fractionalization.[2] Hence, to the extent that a larger government blunts private incentives for productive activity, the behavioral effects are likely to be larger in the United States. Moreover, the United States is much freer to begin with than the Scandinavian countries were in the late 1980s. This leaves much less room for increasing freedom in other dimensions to offset the negative growth effect that would result from a larger government sector.

Against this background there is reason to be concerned about the most recent development and medium-term projections of federal spending levels. U.S. federal spending in 2009 was 24 percent of GDP, which is three percentage points or 14 percent more than the year before, and four percentage points above the 2000–2008 average. In the most recent budget President Obama aspires to reduce the federal spending level by a mere one percentage point to 23 percent of GDP by 2013. Judging from the research reviewed in this essay, this increase in relative government spending is likely to impede economic growth, and hence also impede job creation and recovery from the current crisis.

Notes

Introduction: Why Growth Is Important, and Why Government Size May Matter

1. See for example, Freeman and Schettkat (2005), Davis and Henrekson (2005), and Rogerson (2006).

Chapter 1: How Do We Know If Big Government Is Good or Bad for Growth?

1. For a more in-depth survey of various mechanisms, see Tanzi and Zee (1997).

2. See, for example, Easterly and Rebelo (1993) and Hansson and Henrekson (1994b).

3. See, for example, Solow (1956).

4. It should be noted that this "temporary effect" can easily last for twenty years or more. And if several policy decisions continuously depress private savings, the economy will continuously experience slower growth, holding other factors constant. In fact, Barro and Sala-i-Martin (2004) estimate empirically, based on data at different levels of aggregation, that it takes twenty-five to thirty-five years to eliminate one-half of the deviation from the steady state.

5. See, for example, Romer (1986) and Barro (1990).

6. Here, several studies could be mentioned. A 2004 study by Rodrik and others is often mentioned, and Doucouliagos and Ulubasoglu (2006) and Asoni (2008) provide good overviews.

7. See Carr (1989) and Virén and Koskela (2000).

8. See, for example, Barro (1990) and King and Rebelo (1990). According to King and Rebelo, the welfare cost of a 10 percent increase in the income tax rate can be forty times larger in basic endogenous growth models than in neoclassical growth models.

9. On the latter point, see also Lindbeck (1983).

Chapter 2: What Do Existing Studies Show?

1. In Sweden, for example, most welfare expenditures take place at the local or regional level, and using measures based on central government is therefore highly inappropriate.

2. Similar points have been made by Levine and Renelt (1992), Easterly and Rebelo (1993), and Levine and Zervos (1993).

3. Assuming a normal distribution, most countries can be found in the interval around the mean, plus or minus one standard deviation, and almost all countries (95 percent) can be found within two standard deviations from the mean.

4. As described in Organisation for Economic Co-operation and Development (n.d.).

5. The non-OECD countries added are Chile, Hong Kong, Israel, Korea, Mauritius, Singapore, and Taiwan.

6. The problem in practice is to find good instruments—that is, variables that are not correlated with economic growth but still introduce enough exogenous variation to estimate the relationship. Recently, techniques have been developed that use variables already existing in the dataset as instruments by transforming them in various ways. One such estimator that is currently very popular is the GMM (generalized method of moment) system estimator, which jointly estimates the system with first-difference equations instrumented by lagged levels, and level equations instrumented by first-differences; see Arellano and Bover (1995) and Blundell and Bond (1998). On the other hand, Roodman (2009) has recently cautioned that flawed use of this estimator may produce erroneous results. In the quest for good instruments, Karlsson and Bergh (2008) show that tax credits and basic deductions are, in fact, correlated with government size but uncorrelated with growth, which suggests they can be used as instruments. The problem is that detailed data on deductions and tax credits are available only from 1996, which means that it will take a number of years before a reasonably long time series can be constructed.

Chapter 3: The Growth Effects of Institutional Quality

1. The so-called extreme bounds analysis (EBA) was pioneered by Levine and Renelt (1992) in the context of cross-country growth regressions. The EBA is performed by systematically but mechanically running a large number of regressions with different combinations of conditioning variables among the regressors, to test whether all specifications yield a significant relationship between the main explanatory variable and the dependent variable. An extension of the EBA analysis was suggested by Sala-i-Martin (1997), the basic idea of which is to examine the distribution of coefficient estimates rather than use an absolute criterion of robustness.

2. For more on the resource curse and institutions, see Mehlum and others (2006) and Boschini and others (2007).

3. The correlations shown in figure 3-1 do not change much when using expenditure rather than taxes as a measure of government size, and using government size in 1970 or 2000 rather than average government size during the time period.

4. The southwestern European welfare states refers to Germany, France, Belgium, the Netherlands, Italy, and Switzerland, and the liberal welfare states refers to Australia, the United Kingdom, the United States, and Canada.

5. See, for example, Martin and Schumann (1997) and Strange (1996).

6. See Sinn (1997).

7. See Bergh and Erlingsson (2009), Curzon Price (2008), Rothstein and Lindbom (2004), and Castles (2004).

8. See Koester and Kormendi (1989) for a further discussion of the growth effects of progressivity.

9. Several of these tax reforms have been thoroughly evaluated by academic economists; see, for example, Agell and others (1998) for Sweden and Aarbu and Thoresen (1997) for Norway.

Chapter 4: Deficient Marketization of Household Production in High-Tax Societies

1. See Solow (1957) and Denison (1962).

2. See Freeman and Schettkat (2005) and Olovsson (2009).

3. See SOU (1997:17).

4. Juster and Stafford (1991, 498).

5. This basic insight is important in the theory of optimal taxation. The theoretical results of Kleven and others (2000) and Piggott and Whalley (2001) strongly suggest that the optimal tax structure involves a relatively low tax rate on those market-produced services that could alternatively be produced in the household sector.

6. See Pålsson (1997) and Davis and Henrekson (2005).

7. The marginal tax rate includes the employee's mandatory contributions to social security.

8. Some observers have maintained that the provision of child care and care of the elderly by the public sector offsets most of the services previously produced by the spouse not working in the market. This is a misunderstanding, however, since child care by parents is jointly "produced" with other regular household work, such as shopping, laundry, cleaning, cooking, and so forth.

9. See Henrekson and Johansson (2009) for an in-depth discussion of this effect.

Conclusions and Policy Implications

1. Several such approaches have been used in Denmark, a system sometimes referred to by the term "flexicurity" (Andersen and Haagen Pedersen 2007). This, together with much less stringent employment protection legislation, is arguably an important reason that employment in marginal groups is considerably higher in Denmark than in Sweden despite equally high taxes on labor. The U.S. EITC system and its strong effect on the labor supply of marginal workers, notably single mothers who did not complete high school, is evaluated in Meyer (2007).

2. This is documented by Alesina and Glaeser (2004).

References

Aarbu, Karl Ove, and Thor Olav Thoresen. 1997. The Norwegian Tax Reform: Distributional Effects and the High-Income Response. Discussion Paper No. 207. Oslo: Research Department, Statistics Norway.

Abdiweli, Ali M. 2003. Institutional Differences as Sources of Growth Differences. *Atlantic Economic Journal* 31 (4): 348–62.

Agell, Jonas. 1996. Why Sweden's Welfare State Needed Reform. *Economic Journal* 106 (439): 1760–71.

———, Peter Englund, and Jan Södersten. 1998. *Incentives and Redistribution in the Welfare State—The Swedish Tax Reform.* London: Macmillan.

———, Thomas Lindh, and Henry Ohlsson. 1997. Growth and the Public Sector: A Critical Review Essay. *European Journal of Political Economy* 13 (1): 33–52.

———, Henry Ohlsson, and Peter Skogman Thoursie. 2006. Growth Effects of Government Expenditure and Taxation in Rich Countries: A Comment. *European Economic Review* 50 (1): 211–19.

Alesina, Alberto, and Edward L. Glaeser. 2004. *Fighting Poverty in the U.S. and Europe: A World of Difference.* Oxford: Oxford University Press.

Andersen, Torben, and Lars Haagen Pedersen. 2007. Distribution and Labour Market Incentives in the Welfare State—Danish Experiences. *Swedish Economic Policy Review* 14 (2): 175–214.

Arellano, Manuel, and Olympia Bover. 1995. Another Look at the Instrumental Variable Estimation of Error-Components Models. *Journal of Econometrics* 68 (1): 29–51.

Asoni, Andrea. 2008. Protection of Property Rights and Growth as Political Equilibria. *Journal of Economic Surveys* 22 (5): 953–87.

Ayal, Eliezer B., and Georgios Karras. 1998. Components of Economic Freedom and Growth: An Empirical Study. *Journal of Developing Areas* 32 (3): 327–38.

Barr, Nicholas. 1992. Economic Theory and the Welfare State: A Survey and Interpretation. *Journal of Economic Literature* 30 (2): 741–803.

Barro, Robert J. 1990. Government Spending in a Simple Model of Endogenous Growth. *Journal of Political Economy* 98 (5): 103–25.

———. 1997. *Determinants of Economic Growth: A Cross-Country Empirical Study.* Cambridge, Mass.: MIT Press.

————. 1998a. Notes on Growth Accounting. NBER Working Paper 66546. Cambridge, Mass.: National Bureau of Economic Research.

————. 1998b. Human Capital and Growth in Cross-Country Regressions. Mimeo, Harvard University.

————, and Xavier Sala-i-Martin. 2004. *Economic Growth*. 2nd edition. Cambridge and London: MIT Press.

Becker, Gary S., and Kevin M. Murphy. 1992. The Division of Labor, Coordination Costs, and Knowledge. *Quarterly Journal of Economics* 107 (4): 1137–60.

Bekaert, Geert R., Harvey Campbell, and Christian Lundblad. 2005. Does Financial Liberalization Spur Growth? *Journal of Financial Economics* 77 (1): 3–55.

Berggren, Niclas, and Henrik Jordahl. 2005. Does Free Trade Really Reduce Growth? Further Testing Using the Economic Freedom Index. *Public Choice* 122 (1–2): 99–114.

Bergh, Andreas. 2006. Explaining Welfare State Survival: The Role of Economic Freedom and Globalization. Ratio Working Paper No. 101. Stockholm: Ratio Institute.

————, and Gissur Erlingsson. 2009. Liberalization without Retrenchment: Understanding the Consensus on Swedish Welfare State Reforms. *Scandinavian Political Studies* 32 (1): 71–94.

————, and Martin Karlsson. 2010. Government Size and Growth: Accounting for Economic Freedom and Globalization. *Public Choice* 142 (1–2): 195–213.

Blundell, Richard, and Stephen Bond. 1998. Initial Conditions and Moment Restrictions in Dynamic Panel Data Models. *Journal of Econometrics* 87 (1): 115–43.

Boschini, Anne, Jan Pettersson, and Jesper Roine. 2007. Resource Curse or Not: A Question of Appropriability. *Scandinavian Journal of Economics* 109 (3): 593–617.

Buchanan, James M. 1980. Rent-Seeking and Profit-Seeking. In *Toward a Theory of the Rent-Seeking Society*, ed. James M. Buchanan and Gordon Tullock. College Station, Tex.: Texas A&M University Press.

Cameron, David. 1982. On the Limits of the Public Economy. *Annals of the Academy of Political and Social Science* 459 (1): 46–62.

Carr, Jack L. 1989. Government Size and Economic Growth: A New Framework and Some Evidence from Cross-Section and Time-Series Data: Comment. *American Economic Review* 79 (1): 267–80.

Castles, Francis G. 2004. *The Future of the Welfare State: Crisis Myths and Crisis Realities*. Oxford: Oxford University Press.

Curzon Price, Victoria. 2008. Fiscal Competition and the Optimisation of Tax Revenues for Higher Growth. In *Institutional Competition*, ed. Andreas Bergh and Rolf Höijer. Cheltenham: Edward Elgar.

Dar, A. Atul, and Saleh AmirKhalkhali. 2002. Government Size, Factor Accumulation, and Economic Growth: Evidence from OECD Countries. *Journal of Policy Modeling* 24 (7–8): 679–92.

Davis, Steven J., and Magnus Henrekson. 2005. Tax Effects on Work Activity, Industry Mix and Shadow Economy Size: Evidence from Rich Country Comparisons.

In *Labour Supply and Incentives to Work in Europe*, ed. Ramón Gómez-Salvador, Ana Lamo, Barbara Petrongolo, Melanie Ward, and Etienne Wasmer. Cheltenham: Edward Elgar.

Dawson, John W. 2003. Causality in the Freedom-Growth Relationship. *European Journal of Political Economy* 19 (3): 479–95.

De Haan, Jakob, and Jan-Egbert Sturm. 2000. On the Relationship between Economic Freedom and Economic Growth. *European Journal of Political Economy* 16 (2): 215–41.

De Soto, Hernando. 2000. *The Mystery of Capital: Why Capitalism Triumphs in the West and Fails Everywhere Else*. New York: Basic Books.

Denison, Edward F. 1962. *The Sources of Economic Growth in the United States*. Washington, D.C.: Commission on Economic Development.

Doppelhofer, Gernot, Ronald Miller, and Xavier Sala-i-Martin. 2004. Determinants of Long-Term Growth: A Bayesian Averaging of Classical Estimates (BACE) Approach. *American Economic Review* 94 (4): 813–35.

Doucouliagos, Chris, and Mehmet A. Ulubasoglu. 2006. Economic Freedom and Economic Growth: Does Specification Make a Difference? *European Journal of Political Economy* 22 (1): 60–81.

Dreher, Axel. 2006. Does Globalization Affect Growth? Empirical Evidence from a New Index. *Applied Economics* 38 (10): 1091–110.

Easterly, William, and Sergio Rebelo. 1993. Fiscal Policy and Economic Growth. *Journal of Monetary Economics* 32 (3): 417–58.

Ehrlich, Isaac, and Francis T. Lui. 1999. Bureaucratic Corruption and Endogenous Economic Growth. *Journal of Political Economy* 107 (6): S270–S293.

Feldstein, Martin S. 2006. The Effect of Taxes on Efficiency and Growth. NBER Working Paper No. 12201. Cambridge, Mass.: National Bureau of Economic Research.

Freeman, Richard B. 1995. The Large Welfare State as a System. *American Economic Review* 85 (2): 16–21.

———, and Ronald Schettkat. 2005. Marketization of Household Production and the EU–U.S. Gap in Work. *Economic Policy* 20 (41): 6–50.

Friedman, Thomas. 2005. *The World Is Flat: A Brief History of the Globalized World in the Twenty-first Century*. London: Allen Lane.

Fölster, Stefan, and Magnus Henrekson. 2001. Growth Effects of Government Expenditure and Taxation in Rich Countries. *European Economic Review* 45 (8): 1501–20.

———. 2006. Growth Effects of Government Expenditure and Taxation in Rich Countries: A Reply. *European Economic Review* 50 (1): 219–22.

Gordon, Peter, and Lanlan Wang. 2004. Does Economic Performance Correlate with Big Government? *Econ Journal Watch* 1 (2): 192–221.

Grier, Kevin B., and Gordon Tullock. 1989. An Empirical Analysis of Cross-National Economic Growth, 1951–80. *Journal of Monetary Economics* 24 (2): 259–76.

Gwartney, James D., Randall G. Holcombe, and Robert A. Lawson. 1998. The Scope of Government and the Wealth of Nations. *Cato Journal* 18 (2): 163–90.

———. 2004. Economic Freedom, Institutional Quality, and Cross-Country Differences in Income and Growth. *Cato Journal*, 24: 205-233.

Gwartney, James D., Robert A. Lawson, and Seth Norton. 2008. Economic Freedom of the World: 2008 Annual Report. The Fraser Institute. Data retrieved from www.freetheworld.com.

Hansson, Pär, and Magnus Henrekson. 1994a. A New Framework for Testing the Effect of Government Spending on Growth and Productivity. *Public Choice* 81 (3–4): 381–401.

———. 1994b. What Makes a Country Socially Capable of Catching Up? *Weltwirtschaftliches Archiv* 130 (4): 760–83.

Henrekson, Magnus, and Dan Johansson. 2009. Competencies and Institutions Fostering High-Growth Firms. *Foundations and Trends in Entrepreneurship* 5 (1): 1–80.

Iversen, Torben. 2005. *Capitalism, Democracy and Welfare*. New York: Cambridge University Press.

Jones, Garett, and W. Joel Schneider. 2006. Intelligence, Human Capital, and Economic Growth: A Bayesian Averaging of Classical Estimates (BACE) Approach. *Journal of Economic Growth* 11 (1): 71–93.

Jonung, Christina, and Inga Persson. 1993. Women and Market Work: The Misleading Tale of Participation Rates in International Comparisons. *Work, Employment and Society* 7 (2): 259–74.

Juster, F. Thomas, and Frank P. Stafford. 1991. The Allocation of Time: Empirical Findings, Behavioral Models, and Problems of Measurement. *Journal of Economic Literature* 29 (2): 471–522.

Kaldor, Nicholas. 1966. *Causes of the Slow Rate of Economic Growth of the United Kingdom: An Inaugural Lecture*. Cambridge: Cambridge University Press.

Karlsson, Martin, and Andreas Bergh. 2008. Revisiting the Relation between Government Size and Economic Growth: Accounting for Institutions, Endogeneity and New Data. Paper presented at the meeting of the European Economic Association, Milano, August 27–31.

King, Robert G., and Sergio Rebelo. 1990. Public Policy and Economic Growth: Developing Neoclassical Implications. *Journal of Political Economy* 98 (5): 126–150.

Kleven, Henrik J., Wolfram F. Richter, and Peter B. Sørensen. 2000. Optimal Taxation with Household Production. *Oxford Economic Papers* 52 (3): 584–94.

Knack, Stephen, and Philip Keefer. 1995. Institutions and Economic Performance: Cross-Country Tests Using Alternative Institutional Measures. *Economics and Politics* 7 (3): 207–27.

Koester, Reinhard B., and Roger C. Kormendi. 1989. Taxation, Aggregate Activity and Economic Growth: Cross-Country Evidence on Some Supply-Side Hypotheses. *Economic Inquiry* 27 (3): 367–86.

Kristov, Lorenzo, Peter H. Lindert, and Robert McClelland. 1992. Pressure Groups and Redistribution. *Journal of Public Economics* 48 (2): 135–63.

Landau, David. 1983. Government Expenditure and Economic Growth: A Cross-Country Study. *Southern Economic Journal* 49 (3): 783–92

Leamer, Edward. 2007. A Flat World, a Level Playing Field, a Small World After All, or None of the Above? A Review of Thomas L. Friedman's *The World Is Flat. Journal of Economic Literature* 45 (1): 83–126.

Levine, Ross, and David Renelt. 1992. A Sensitivity Analysis of Cross-Country Growth Regressions. *American Economic Review* 82 (4): 942–63.

Levine, Ross, and Sara J. Zervos. 1993. What We Have Learned About Policy and Growth from Cross-Country Regressions. *American Economic Review* 83 (2): 426–30.

Lindbeck, Assar. 1982. Tax Effects versus Budget Effects on Labor Supply. *Economic Inquiry* 20 (3): 473–89.

———. 1983. Budget Expansion and Cost Inflation. *American Economic Review* 73 (2): 285–96.

Lindert, Peter H. 2003. Why the Welfare State Looks Like a Free Lunch. NBER Working Paper 9869. Cambridge, Mass.: National Bureau of Economic Research.

———. 2004. *Growing Public*. Cambridge: Cambridge University Press.

Loayza, Norman V., and Romain Ranciere. 2006. Financial Development, Financial Fragility, and Growth. *Journal of Money, Credit, and Banking* 38 (4): 1051–76.

Lucas, Robert E. 1988. On the Mechanics of Economic Development. *Journal of Monetary Economics* 22 (1): 3–42.

Madrick, Jeff. 2009. *The Case for Big Government*. Princeton, N.J.: Princeton University Press.

Marlow, Michael L. 1986. Private Sector Shrinkage and the Growth of Industrialized Economies. *Public Choice* 49 (2): 143–54.

Martin, Hans-Peter, and Harald Schumann. 1997. *The Global Trap: Globalization and the Assault on Prosperity and Democracy*. London, New York: Zed Books.

Mehlum, Halvor, Karl Moene, and Ragnar Torvik. 2006. Cursed by Resources or Institutions? *World Economy* 29 (8): 1117–31.

Meyer, Bruce D. 2007. The US Earned Income Tax Credit, Its Effects, and Possible Reforms. *Swedish Economic Policy Review* 14 (2): 55–80.

Myrdal, Gunnar. 1960. *Beyond the Welfare State*. New Haven, Conn.: Yale University Press.

Nelson, Michael, A., and Ram D. Singh. 1998. Democracy, Economic Freedom, Fiscal Policy, and Growth in LDCs: A Fresh Look. *Economic Development and Cultural Change* 46 (3): 677–96.

North, Douglass C. 1987. Institutions, Transaction Costs and Economic Growth. *Economic Inquiry* 25 (3): 419–28.

Okun, Arthur M. 1975. *Equality and Efficiency: The Big Tradeoff*. Washington, D.C.: Brookings Institution.

Olovsson, Conny. 2009. Why Do Europeans Work So Little? *International Economic Review* 50 (1): 39–61.

Olson, Mancur. 1982. *The Rise and Decline of Nations: Economic Growth, Stagflation, and Social Rigidities.* New Haven, Conn.: Yale University Press.

Organisation for Economic Co-operation and Development (n.d.). About OECD. http://www.oecd.org/pages/0,3417,en_36734052_36734103_1_1_1_1_1,00.html (accessed January 13, 2010).

Pålsson, Anne-Marie. 1997. Taxation and the Market for Domestic Services. In *Economics of the Family and Family Policies*, ed. Inga Persson and Christina Jonung. London: Routledge.

Piggott, John, and John Whalley. 2001. VAT Base Broadening, Self Supply, and the Informal Sector. *American Economic Review* 91 (4): 1084–94.

Plosser, Charles I. 1992. The Search for Growth. In *Policies for Long-Run Economic Growth: A Symposium Sponsored by the Federal Reserve Bank of Kansas City.* Jackson Hole, Wyoming, August 27–29. Kansas City: Federal Reserve Bank of Kansas City.

Pritchett, Lant, and Lawrence H. Summers. 1996. Wealthier Is Healthier. *Journal of Human Resources* 31 (4): 841–68.

Rodriguez, Enrique. 1981. *Den svenska skattehistorien.* Lund: Liber Läromedel.

Rodrik, Dani, Arvind Subramanian, and Francesco Trebbi. 2004. Institutions Rule: The Primacy of Institutions over Geography and Integration in Economic Development. *Journal of Economic Growth* 9 (2): 131–65.

Rogerson, Richard. 2006. Understanding Differences in Hours Worked. *Review of Economic Dynamics* 9 (3): 365–409.

Romer, Paul M. 1986. Increasing Returns and Long-Run Growth. *Journal of Political Economy* 94 (5): 1002–37.

Romero-Avila, Diego, and Rolf Strauch. 2008. Public Finances and Long-Term Growth in Europe: Evidence from a Panel Data Analysis. *European Journal of Political Economy* 24 (1): 172–91.

Roodman, David. 2009. A Note on the Theme of Too Many Instruments. *Oxford Bulletin of Economics and Statistics* 71 (1): 135–58.

Rosen, Sherwin. 1983. Specialization and Human Capital. *Journal of Labor Economics* 1 (1): 43–49.

Rosling, Hans. 2010. Gapminder website, http://www.gapminder.org/ (accessed January 1, 2010).

Rothstein, Bo, and Anders Lindbom. 2004. The Mysterious Survival of the Scandinavian Welfare States. Paper presented at the annual meeting of the American Political Science Association, Chicago.

Sala-i-Martin, Xavier. 1997. I Just Ran 2 Million Regressions. *American Economic Review* 87 (2): 178–83.

Sanandaji, Tino, and Fabian Wallen. 2009. Allocation of Time and Leisure in Europe and the U.S. Mimeo, University of Chicago and the Confederation of Swedish Enterprise, Stockholm.

Saunders, Peter. 1986. What Can We Learn from International Comparisons of Public Sector Size and Economic Performance? *European Sociological Review* 2 (1): 52–60.

———. 1988. Private Sector Shrinkage and the Growth of Industrialized Economies: Comment. *Public Choice* 58 (3): 277–84.

Schmid, Günther. 2008. *Full Employment in Europe—Managing Labour Market Transitions and Risks*. Cheltenham: Edward Elgar.

Sinn, Hans-Werner. 1997. The Selection Principle and Market Failure in Systems Competition. *Journal of Public Economics* 66 (2): 247–74.

Smith, Adam. 1776 [1965]. *The Wealth of Nations*. New York: Modern Library.

Solow, Robert M. 1956. A Contribution to the Theory of Economic Growth. *Quarterly Journal of Economics* 70 (1): 65–94.

———. 1957. Technical Change and the Aggregate Production Function. *Review of Economics and Statistics* 39 (3): 312–20.

SOU 1997:17. *Skatter, Tjänster och Sysselsättning*. Final report of the Swedish Government Inquiry on the Taxation of Services. Stockholm: Ministry of Finance.

Stevenson, Betsey, and Justin Wolfers. 2008. Economic Growth and Subjective Well-Being: Reassessing the Easterlin Paradox. *Brookings Papers on Economic Activity* 1: 1–87.

Strange, Susan. 1996. *The Retreat of the State: The Diffusion of Power in the World Economy*. Cambridge: Cambridge University Press.

Sturm, Jan-Egbert, and Jakob De Haan. 2001. How Robust is the Relationship between Economic Freedom and Economic Growth? *Applied Economics* 33 (7): 839–44.

Tanzi, Vito, and Ludger Schuknecht. 1997. Reconsidering the Fiscal Role of Government: The International Perspective. *American Economic Review* 87 (1): 164–68.

———, and Howell H. Zee. 1997. Fiscal Policy and Long-Run Growth. *IMF Staff Papers* 44 (2): 179–209.

Virén, Matti, and Erkki Koskela. 2000. Is There a Laffer Curve between Aggregate Output and Public Sector Employment? *Empirical Economics* 25 (4): 605–21.

Widmalm, Frida. 2001. Tax Structure and Growth: Are Some Taxes Better than Others? *Public Choice* 107 (3–4): 199–219.

Yang, Benhua. 2008. FDI and Growth: A Varying Relationship Across Regions and Over Time. *Applied Economics Letters* 15 (2): 105–8.

About the Authors

Andreas Bergh has a PhD from Lund University, Sweden, and was a visiting scholar at Harvard University in 2004. In 2005, he became a research fellow at the Ratio Institute in Stockholm, where he researches welfare state reform and institutional economics. In 2010, Bergh became affiliated with the Research Institute of Industrial Economics in Stockholm.

Magnus Henrekson is president of the Research Institute of Industrial Economics, Stockholm. Until 2009, he was Jacob Wallenberg Professor of Economics at the Stockholm School of Economics. In recent years, his research has focused on institutional determinants of entrepreneurial activity and explanations for cross-country differences in economic performance.

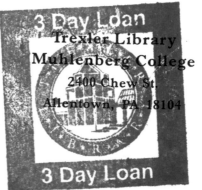